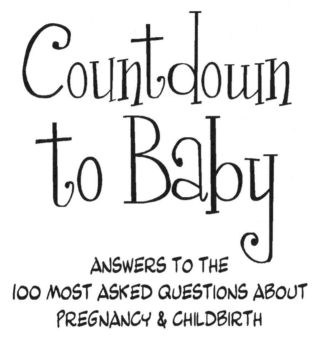

Countdown to Baby

ANSWERS TO THE 100 MOST ASKED QUESTIONS ABOUT PREGNANCY & CHILDBIRTH

SUSAN WARHUS, M.D.

Addicus Books
Omaha, Nebraska

An Addicus Nonfiction Book

ISBN# 1-886039-68-2

Cover design by Peri Poloni
Illustrations by Jack Kusler

This book is not intended to serve as a substitute for a physician nor is it the author's intent to give medical advice contrary to that of an attending physician.

Library of Congress Cataloging-in-Publication Data

Warhus, Susan P., 1955-
    Countdown to baby : answers to the 100 most asked questions about pregnancy and childbirth / Susan P. Warhus.
        p. cm.
    ISBN 1-886039-68-2
    1. Pregnancy—Popular works. 2. Pregnancy—Miscellanea. 3. Childbirth—Popular works. 4. Childbirth—Miscellanea. I. Title.
    RG551.W374 2003
    618.2—dc22   2003016803

Addicus Books, Inc.
P.O. Box 45327
Omaha, Nebraska 68145
www.AddicusBooks.com
Printed in the United States of America
10 9 8 7 6 5 4 3 2 1

To all the women whose prenatal care and childbirth experience I've had the honor of sharing. Thank you for allowing me to participate in such a magical time in your lives.

Contents

vii

viii

Acknowledgments

I would like to thank my wonderful husband Larry for always being my "pillar of strength" and loving partner in life. I know that I am blessed to share my life with you. I also thank my awesome son Kevin. You are a bright, great kid. I appreciate both of you for being so understanding and patient when I was "always on the computer."

A huge thanks to Jennifer, who is the most amazing nurse I've ever known. I appreciate your efforts to make this book a great success. I value you as a supportive and caring friend.

I also acknowledge my former partner Mary Ellen, an incredible doctor, who took the time out of her insanely busy schedule to review this manuscript for accuracy and completeness. Thanks, also, to my favorite midwife and new mother, Ana, for providing special insights and information for this book.

I've always enjoyed working with the outstanding professionals at Scottsdale Healthcare Women's Center, both the administrative and nursing staff. Thank you for supporting my goal to pursue women's health issues and patient education.

Finally, I would like to thank the staff at Addicus Books. Thank you, especially, to Rod and Susan for believing in me and guiding me through this process when others would not take the chance with a first-time author.

Introduction

I was motivated to write this book by my own experiences, both personal and professional. First, my own pregnancy and childbirth did not go the way I had hoped. I happened to be finishing medical school at the time of my delivery. (In fact, I actually missed the graduation ceremony because I was in the hospital.) I thought I knew a lot more about labor and delivery than I really did. I was disappointed and felt that I had been misled about the pain of childbirth, the role of my own physician, and several complications that eventually required me to have a Cesarean section. I hope I can help you avoid some of those same pitfalls.

As a doctor, it's my goal to provide you with the best information available so that you can have the most rewarding pregnancy and childbirth experience. I am a board-certified OB/GYN physician and have delivered more than 3,000 babies. During my almost fifteen years in clinical practice, I provided medical care to thousands of pregnant women. Most of these patients already owned one of those large reference books on pregnancy. However, during their prenatal visits, they always had many additional questions and concerns to discuss with me. I noticed that the same questions were being asked over and over again. I decided to keep a list of the most common questions, and that process was the genesis of this book. It focuses on the pregnant woman's most frequently asked questions and her top concerns. I've tried to answer the questions fully, yet concisely.

I hope that you enjoy this book and find it helpful. I am pleased to be able to offer help during this special time in your life. I wish you all the best on your continued journey toward motherhood. Your life is about to miraculously change forever.

Part I
First Trimester

1

Getting Organized

Congratulations, you're pregnant! What an exciting time in your life! Now that you're pregnant, you have lots of things on your mind and many things to do. Be assured that it is perfectly normal to experience a wide range of emotions. Some days you may be bursting with delight and excitement; at other times you may feel frightened and overwhelmed. You can reduce some of the stress you might be feeling by getting organized and making some important decisions. Your top priority right now is to establish excellent prenatal care for yourself and your unborn baby. You need to find the best doctor (or midwife) to care for you during your pregnancy and upcoming delivery. You also need to review diet, exercise, and other lifestyle habits that are important to maintain during your pregnancy.

You are about to embark on your amazing journey toward motherhood, and your life will never again be quite the same. Best wishes to you during your pregnancy. It is such a special time.

1. How is my due date calculated?

Your due date is calculated based on the first day of your last menstrual cycle. That's why it's important to keep a record of your periods when you are trying to get pregnant. You become pregnant when your body is ovulating. *Ovulation* is the releasing of an egg from one of your ovaries. The egg can only be fertilized within twenty-four to thirty-six hours of ovulation. If you have intercourse during ovulation time, there is a good chance that one of the millions of sperm released during your partner's ejaculation will fertilize your egg. Most women cycle approximately every 28 days and ovulate on or about day 14. The easiest way to determine your menstrual or fertility cycle is to begin counting on the first day of your period; this is day one. Continue to count each day until you reach day 14. For most women, day 14 is ovulation day and the most likely day for you to become pregnant. After day 14, continue to count each day. If you are pregnant, you won't have another period. If you are not pregnant, continue to count (usually until about day 28) until your next period begins and the cycle starts all over again with day one.

The due date of a full-term pregnancy is based on 40 weeks from the first day of your last period. Another way of looking at it is to say that your due date is about 38 weeks after conception. However, the medical profession uses the 40 weeks from your last period method. Those little gestational wheels used to calculate due dates that you see in your doctor's office are based on the same 40-week term method. Ask your doctor to show you how it works.

In some cases, it may be difficult to determine your due date. Perhaps you don't remember when your last period was, or maybe your periods are irregular. In these cases, the doctor will often order an ultrasound to assist in determining the due date.

2. When should I tell my family and friends that I am pregnant?

The decision to tell others about your pregnancy is entirely up to you. Most women immediately share the news with spouse, partner, or a close friend. This is usually a good idea because it enables you to discuss your excitement and share your concerns with a close and supportive person in your life. However, before you announce the big news to your entire family and all your friends, and coworkers, you may want to consider a few important issues.

Many women prefer to know that the fetus is viable before telling others. This may be especially true if you have had miscarriages or ectopic pregnancies in the past. Once you have heard or seen the fetal heartbeat, there is a greater than 95 percent chance that the fetus will not miscarry. Waiting until you have that reassurance allows you to avoid the difficulty and sadness of having to announce that a miscarriage has occurred.

Some women, especially those over thirty-five, prefer to know that the baby's genetic makeup is normal prior to announcing news of their pregnancy. (If you are age thirty-five or older, your baby has a slightly increased chance of having genetic abnormalities.) If test results show a genetic abnormality, the woman has the option to confidentially terminate her pregnancy.

On the other hand, some women enjoy sharing the big news with everyone right away. By immediately announcing your pregnancy to your group of family and friends, you are able to celebrate your happiness with all of them. Should a miscarriage or problem occur, you would also receive sympathy and encouragement from a large support system.

Once the news of your pregnancy becomes widespread, prepare yourself for a barrage of advice, warnings, and stories. When it comes to pregnancy and childbirth, just about every woman considers herself an expert and has a story to tell. Even though their comments are made out of love and concern for you, eventually these remarks may cause you undue worry and concern. Perhaps your well-intentioned friend doesn't remember the entire story, or maybe technology has changed since a particular incident happened. The important thing for you to do is establish a close relationship with a caring and communicative doctor. Your health provider, who knows you and your situation, is best qualified to address your concerns and questions. Your doctor is there to care for you and also to comfort and reassure you through the entire pregnancy and childbirth experience.

3. What changes in my diet, exercise, and lifestyle should I make?

In a perfect world, you would maintain an ideal, healthy lifestyle and have absolutely no vices or bad habits. That would mean that you don't smoke and you've avoided all alcohol, medication, and drug use. It would also mean that you eat a well-balanced diet, exercise in moderation two to three times each week, and take one prenatal vitamin per day. Honestly, that is rarely the situation. Once you find out that you're pregnant, immediately stop the use of all tobacco, alcohol, or drugs and do your best to eat a healthy diet. If you are already participating in an exercise program, it's fine to continue. However, most experts agree that pregnancy is not a good time to begin a vigorous exercise routine, because your body is already going through so many other important changes. If you were taking prenatal vitamins prior to becoming pregnant, it's fine to continue. Otherwise, they will be prescribed for you at your first prenatal visit.

Prior to finding out that you are pregnant, you may have done some things that are now causing you anxiety and concern. For example, perhaps you had a couple of alcoholic beverages, smoked cigarettes, or used certain types of medication. It's important to let your doctor know this during your first prenatal visit. That's because the doctor may want to order an ultrasound or watch your pregnancy more closely for signs of possible miscarriage.

Many studies have indicated that use of alcohol, tobacco, or drugs in the first days of pregnancy usually results in an "all or nothing" outcome. That means it is possible that the embryo could suffer a devastating blow from those unhealthy toxins, and a miscarriage could result. However it is more common that absolutely nothing happens to the embryo because it has not yet become established enough with your own blood supply. It is extremely reassuring to know that in these types of circumstances, the embryo is rarely injured.

For the remainder of your pregnancy, as baby's blood supply becomes more incorporated with your own, it is essential for baby's growth and development that you maintain healthy lifestyle habits.

Avoid Tobacco, Alcohol, Drugs

These toxins can be damaging to you and especially devastating to your fetus. Smoking can cause the following complications:

- low birth weight
- preterm birth
- vaginal bleeding
- placental abruption (placenta separates from uterus)

These are all harmful to the fetus. I've heard women say, "I'm going to keep smoking because I want to deliver a small baby. That way, delivery won't be so painful." The truth is, smoking during pregnancy doesn't make the baby petite; it can seriously influence the fetus's growth pattern and blood supply. Usually the fetal head continues to grow normally while the growth of the rest of the fetus's body is slowed. The medical term for this is *intrauterine growth retardation (IUGR)*. Quitting smoking completely is best. If you can't quit smoking entirely, then cut back to as few cigarettes as possible. Talk to your doctor for advice and options.

Alcohol can cause the following complications:

- lowered heart rate for you and the baby
- fetal alcohol syndrome
- mental retardation
- various physical abnormalities

Since it is unknown exactly how much alcohol causes fetal alcohol syndrome, the safest course is not to consume any alcohol at all during pregnancy. Use of other drugs can cause the following complications:

- vaginal bleeding
- placental abruption (placenta separates from uterus)
- preterm birth
- low birth weight
- major birth defects
- drug dependency in baby (irritable, crying baby)
- fetal death

If you have a drug problem, please confide in your doctor to get help.

Diet

Especially during the first trimester, it is normal not to feel very hungry. Sometimes you may have cravings for certain foods. It is important to drink eight glasses of water each day and attempt to make healthy food choices. Your fetus needs certain nutrients to grow and develop properly. The foods that you eat are the fetus's primary source of vitamins and minerals. It's best to follow a well-balanced food plan. The USDA food pyramid recommends these daily servings during pregnancy:

Recommended Food and Servings during Pregnancy

Food Group	Daily Number of Servings
Bread/cereal/rice/pasta	9
Vegetable	4
Fruit	3
Meat/poultry/fish/dry beans/eggs/nuts	3
Milk/yogurt/cheese	3

It is also a good idea to reduce your intake of foods loaded with sugar, such as soda, cakes, pies, ice cream, and candy. Most pregnant women prefer eating five or six small meals each day rather than the traditional three meals per day. Eating small, frequent meals helps to prevent heartburn and indigestion because your stomach doesn't get so full. Also, your sugar levels stay more even, so you feel better. Remember to consume an additional 300 calories per day over your usual prepregnancy calorie intake.

During pregnancy it is best to avoid eating raw fish or raw meat because of their potential for harboring bacteria or parasites. In the worst case, these organisms could cause harm to the fetus. In other cases, they could cause you to have nausea, vomiting, and diarrhea. Not only is this miserable for you, but it may lead to dehydration and reduced nutrition for the fetus.

Certain cooked fish, including shark, swordfish, king mackerel, and tuna, could contain high levels of mercury that may lead to damage of the nervous system. They should be avoided.

Brie, feta, Camembert, and other soft cheeses are at high risk for containing bacteria called *listeria*. According to the FDA, listeria can pose serious health risks for pregnant women.

Exercise

Exercise during pregnancy can be helpful. However, if you are not used to exercising, be sure to begin cautiously and slowly. If you already have an established exercise routine, you may continue with it, keeping the following considerations in mind.

Listen to your body and don't overdo it. Talk with your doctor to make sure he or she has no objections to your participation in pregnancy-safe exercises. If you have certain health conditions such as high blood pressure, preterm labor, or vaginal bleeding, your doctor may advise against exercise.

Exercise Tips during Pregnancy

Remember:	Because:
Keep your maximum heart rate below 150 beats per minute	Fetus's heart rate increases as your does
Drink lots of water, fluids	Dehydration contributes to preterm labor
Wear a supportive bra	Growing changing breasts need extra support
Avoid being flat on back after 20 weeks	Circulation to baby reduced by growing uterus
Avoid high-impact, jumpy, jarring motions	Violent motions could result in injury
Go walking, swimming, stationary biking	These are examples of great, safe exercises
Avoid downhill racing, skating, horseback riding	These are examples of dangerous exercises
STOP! If bleeding, contractions, dizziness, heart racing	Warning signs to rest and call doctor

Assuming your doctor has cleared you for a pregnancy exercise program, you will begin to notice many benefits. Exercise will give you more energy, decrease aches and discomforts, decrease bloating, make you feel stronger, and help you sleep better. Overall, you should feel much better about your body and yourself.

4. How do I select the best doctor to deliver my baby?

The best way to find a good doctor is through word of mouth. Ask your friends, coworkers, and neighbors for recommendations. If you are new to the community, call a local hospital's labor and delivery department and ask the nurses whom they recommend. Once you have gathered a list of names, you need to narrow it down. Unfortunately in today's society, your insurance company may dictate which doctors and which hospitals you may select, so be sure to check your insurance book listing. You may also narrow the list by location or by gender of the doctor, if you desire.

When you have just two or three names, you may select one from that list to become your doctor and set up your first prenatal appointment. When calling to schedule your first appointment, have your calendar handy, your health insurance card available, and the date of your last menstrual period, if known.

If you'd rather interview several doctors before narrowing your list, that can sometimes be arranged. Some doctors provide an OB consultation appointment at no charge. Others charge a regular office visit fee. Here are some examples of questions that you may want to ask when selecting your OB/GYN physician.

OB/GYN Selection Process Questions

Suggested Questions	Good Answers	Because the Doctor...
Are you board-certified?	yes	Possesses proper level of training or knowledge
How many hospitals do you go to?	1 or 2	Can be more focused on patients
How many deliveries do you do?	14-18 per month	Keeps skills sharp, but is not overwhelmed
What is your C-section rate?	17-25%	Is within the national average of 23%
Can I meet your partners?	yes	May have partner do your delivery
Can you be reached after hours	yes	Has a twenty-four-hour service
What do you use for labor pain?	open-minded	Accommodates your plan for pain relief

While the answers to the questions are important, the most crucial point is that you feel comfortable with the doctor. You need to feel that the doctor you select is competent, trustworthy, and open to communication.

Occasionally, after establishing care with the physician, you may decide that you don't feel comfortable with the physician after all. If this occurs, evaluate the situation thoroughly and seriously consider changing physicians. After all, your pregnancy and the birth of your baby are very special times in your life. You deserve to have the best experience possible.

5. What about having a midwife deliver my baby?

Many pregnant women like the idea of being delivered by a midwife. They envision an understanding, gentle, and well-trained woman who will take extra care and time with them during their pregnancy and delivery. Midwives are more likely to be at your side during the entire labor process. They tend to emphasize emotional and physical support in a nurturing environment.

However, midwives are not suitable for every patient. Certain factors regarding your heath and medical history should be considered to determine whether a midwife is a good choice for you. For example, can you answer "yes" to these questions?

- Are you a low-risk patient without any known medical or pregnancy-related problems?
- Have you previously delivered a baby vaginally without any complications?
- Does your hospital permit midwives to practice there?
- Will your insurance pay for a midwife's services?

If you answered yes to all the questions, using a midwife may be a consideration for you. Like physicians, midwives provide prenatal care, manage and evaluate your progress in labor, and deliver your baby.

Unlike physicians, midwives do not have the training to care for patients with medical conditions or complicated pregnancies. Therefore, if you are diabetic, are carrying multiple fetuses, have high blood pressure, or have other medical conditions, you should be under the care of a physician. Midwives do not have the skills to perform deliveries that require additional expertise, such as vacuum, forceps, or C-section deliveries. If you have previously had a normal vaginal delivery, a midwife provides you with a safe alternative to a physician. That's because once you have delivered vaginally, you will most likely be able to deliver vaginally again without complications. However, if this is your first baby or you have only delivered by C-section in the past, you have what is referred to as an "unproven pelvis." It's unknown whether or not you can safely deliver vaginally. Also, if you had a C-section in the past, there is a small chance that your old uterine scar could rupture during labor. In either case, your chances for requiring the technical expertise of a physician are greater than those of a woman who has delivered vaginally in the past. That's why a physician is recommended over a midwife in such cases.

Assuming that a midwife is still a good option for you, be sure to check with your hospital and health insurance provider to ensure that midwife services are allowed and covered.

When selecting a midwife, you should have an understanding about the different kinds of midwives. Their education and training can vary greatly. In the United States, the two main categories of midwives are the Certified Nurse-Midwife (CNM) and the lay (direct-entry) midwife.

Note that the CNM has the best qualifications. She is a licensed and registered nurse with additional midwifery graduate school training. Almost 100 percent of her deliveries occur in the hospital setting with a physician as backup in case of emergencies. The CNM is also a GYN nurse practitioner, so she is able to provide routine care for you when you are not pregnant, including such things as taking Pap smears, prescribing contraception, and treating vaginal infections.

Categories of Midwives

	Certified Nurse-Midwife	Lay Midwife
Registered nurse	Yes	No
State license	Yes	No
Education	College, master's level	Varies
Doctor backup	Yes	Varies
Location of delivery	Hospital	Home
Hospital privileges	Yes	No
GYN abilities	Yes	No

The lay midwife is not a nurse or nurse practitioner. Her education and training can vary widely. Typically, lay midwives learn their craft by apprenticing under other lay midwives. Some lay midwives are members of a lay midwife association and abide by their standards and practices. Most lay midwife deliveries are done in the home setting.

It is a great safety measure to deliver in a hospital and to have a backup doctor available in the rare case of emergencies. In the case of fetal distress or other complications beyond the scope of the CNM's practice, she would call her backup physician for assistance. The doctor would assess the situation and either try for a vaginal delivery or proceed directly with a C-section. Although midwives are not qualified to perform C-sections, some CNMs are trained to assist the physician with a C-section.

Some doctors hire midwives (usually CNMs) to work in their offices, assist, and perform deliveries. This is a good option because the doctor and midwife. Participate in the patient's care, and they function together as a team.

2

First Prenatal Visits

By the time you have your first prenatal visit, you've probably known about your pregnancy for several weeks. This is often a time of great excitement and anticipation. You are probably eager to officially begin your prenatal care and ensure that everything is fine. It's not uncommon to have a lot of concerns about the pregnancy and the changes happening to your body. It's always a good idea to take along a list of your questions and concerns to this first visit, as well as to the ones that follow. A list comes in handy in case other issues distract you during your visits.

You may already be an established patient of the obstetrician's medical practice and be familiar with the staff and the office procedures. However, if you are new to the practice, be sure that you are introduced to the key medical staff, are given important phone numbers (for appointments, emergencies, and after-hour calls), and have a general understanding of how the office works. Often new patients receive this information in the form of a "Welcome to Our Practice" brochure or kit.

1. When should I schedule my first prenatal visit?

Ideally, your first prenatal visit should be scheduled approximately six to eight weeks after your last period. This timing is early enough to discuss how the pregnancy may influence any medical conditions or problems that you already are known to have. For example, if you are a known diabetic or have a thyroid disorder, your medication may require adjustment due to the pregnancy. Six to eight weeks into the pregnancy is also a good time to begin taking your prenatal vitamins, so they are usually prescribed at this visit. This visit's timing also provides ample time to consider and arrange for genetic evaluation of the fetus if that is indicated. (The actual testing is generally performed at between 10 and 16 weeks.) If you experience bleeding or cramping prior to your scheduled first visit, see your doctor immediately. These could be warning signs of possible miscarriage or ectopic pregnancy.

It can be helpful to have a companion accompany you for your first prenatal visit, especially if this is your first time going to the office. It's good to hear your partner's opinion of the medical staff and facility. If you are feeling overwhelmed, your partner may be able to make observations or ask relevant questions. Also, if you have important decisions to make about issues such as fetal genetic evaluation, repeat Cesarean section, or permanent sterilization, your partner can also receive information and take part in the discussion.

On the other hand, some women prefer to keep certain aspects of their medical histories private and confidential. For example, you may wish to keep a herpes diagnosis or a past abortion secret from a family member or friend. Similarly, some women prefer privacy and don't want their companions to view their partially clothed bodies during the physical examination. Naturally, you may ask your loved one to leave during these times, or you may prefer that he or she accompany you at a later visit, when these types of examinations or discussions will not be held.

Your first prenatal visit will almost certainly be the longest of all the prenatal visits. If you plan to take your spouse, partner, or close friend along, let him or her know that the visit may last one to two hours.

2.   What is a medical history interview?

Once you have scheduled your first prenatal visit, many doctors will mail you a lengthy medical history health questionnaire. They request that you complete it and bring it with you to the first prenatal visit. If that has not been done, you will probably be asked to come early to fill out the information in the doctor's waiting area. While you are doing this, the medical assistant will often ask you for a urine sample to confirm a positive pregnancy test before proceeding any further with the visit.

After the pregnancy has been confirmed, you are called back into an interview room. The purpose of this interview is to obtain a very detailed history of your past and present medical conditions. Your doctor or your doctor's nurse practitioner will conduct the interview and will discuss a number of issues.

- *Due Date:* The provider will first determine your due date based on the date of your last period. If there is confusion about your dates, an ultrasound may be ordered and performed as soon as possible.
- *Current Problems:* The interviewer will ask if you are having any problems, especially bleeding, cramping, or pain.
- *Past Pregnancies:* The doctor or nurse practitioner will want to know of any major problems or complications you had with past pregnancies. Be sure to mention difficulties with vaginal deliveries or Cesarean sections.
- *Prior Cesarean Section:* If you have had a prior Cesarean section (C-section), the interviewer will discuss the options of a repeat C-section versus a trial of *vaginal birth after C-section (VBAC)*. If you desire a repeat C-section, you will be asked whether you want permanent sterilization, also known as having your tubes tied.
- *Medical Conditions:* The physician or nurse practitioner with whom you are speaking will ask about your current

medications and any known diseases, surgeries, serious infections, or allergies. It is extremely important to mention any history of diabetes, high blood pressure, anemia, heart disease, or other serious conditions. You should also let your health professional know about any of the following issues or conditions:

- *Herpes:* If you have a lesion at time of delivery, a C-section is usually recommended to avoid lesion contact with the baby. Herpes infection in newborns can be life-threatening.
- *HIV:* If you are known to be HIV positive, medication given to you during your pregnancy can greatly reduce the chance of the baby acquiring the virus.
- *Over Age Thirty-Five at Time of Delivery:* If you will be thirty-five or older at the time of delivery, you and the interviewer will discuss the possibility of genetic counseling and testing.
- *Family History:* The interviewer will ask whether you have a family history of any particular disease or genetic abnormality. If you do, be prepared to provide the details.
- *Lifestyle Habits:* The practitioner will address the issues of nutrition, exercise, and tobacco, alcohol, and drug use.
- *Domestic Violence:* If there is a past history of domestic violence or a current threat to you and your unborn baby, the practitioner needs to know. Take him or her into your confidence.

During this detailed discussion, be sure to tell your health provider if you have additional medical problems or concerns.

After you have finished the conversation, the health provider will probably leave the room and give you privacy to change into a patient examination gown. The provider will return shortly to conduct a thorough physical examination.

3. Will I be able to hear the baby's heartbeat at this visit?

Assuming that your first prenatal visit occurs during the first 6 to 8 weeks of pregnancy, it will be too early to hear the baby's heartbeat. Many women feel very disappointed when they are given this news. With a special listening device called a Doptone, the fetal heartbeat is usually heard at about 10 to 12 weeks. Hearing the fetal heartbeat will likely be the highlight of your second prenatal visit.

4. What is involved in the physical examination?

You will probably be relieved to know that the first prenatal visit is the only visit that involves the detailed physical examination outlined in the table here. Unless there is a problem such as bleeding, infection, pain, or premature labor, you will probably not have any further pelvic examinations until about 36 weeks.

At the conclusion of your physical examination and lab testing, your health provider will give you any needed prescriptions, including one for prenatal vitamins. Before you leave, make sure all of your concerns have been addressed. Typically, you will be asked to return for your next prenatal visit in about four weeks.

5. When should I begin prenatal vitamins?

At the end of your first prenatal visit, the doctor or nurse practitioner will give you samples of or a prescription for prenatal vitamins. Unless you are suffering from extreme morning sickness, it is a good idea to begin the vitamins immediately. That's because many pregnant women (or women in general, for that matter) don't always eat a well-balanced diet. A good prenatal vitamin will give you the extra supplements that you may not get from your diet. Ideally, you should begin your prenatal vitamin several months before you even become pregnant.

Testing Done at First Prenatal Visit

Exam/Test	Checking/Evaluating	Important Because...
Physical Exam	Heart, lungs, breasts, other organs	Looks for disease or abnormalities that could influence the pregnancy
Pelvic Exam	Uterus and cervix	Determines size of uterus, ensures cervix is closed and not bleeding
	Pap smear	Detects abnormal cells on cervix
	GC and chlamydia	Checks for infection; may need antibiotics
Blood Work	Blood type	Establishes blood type in case you need transfusion
	Immunity to rubella status (German measles)	Checks rubella status; if not immune, avoid people with measles, get vaccination after delivery
	Anemia	Determines whether iron or other supplements are needed
	Rh status	Determines status; may need RhoGAM
	Antibody screen	Determines status; may need special testing
	Syphilis	Checks for infection; may need antibiotics
	HIV	Determines status; may require medication
Urine Analysis	Presence of bacteria	Checks if present; may need antibiotics
	Presence of protein	Checks if present; may be indicator of kidney disease
	Presence of sugar	Checks if present; sometimes an indicator of diabetes

More important is the issue of folic acid. All prenatal vitamins now contain between 0.4 and 1.0 mg of folic acid. When you take folic acid before you become pregnant and also during your first few months of pregnancy, you can help prevent the risk of neural tube birth defects. A neural tube birth defect is an abnormality in which the spine or brain does not close properly. This type of birth defect can be quite serious and may result in either severe disability or even death for the baby. Fortunately, neural tube defects are extremely rare. By taking your prenatal vitamin with folic acid, you can reduce the chances even more.

Your body needs extra iron and calcium when you are pregnant or breast-feeding. The doctor will check your blood sample in the lab and will also discuss your diet. Depending on these results, your health provider may recommend supplemental iron or calcium. Calcium totaling 1,200 milligrams each day is recommended while pregnant or breast-feeding. If you are not getting that much from your diet, speak with your physician about calcium supplements.

All prenatal vitamins are basically the same in their nutritional content. However, they do vary according to flavor, size, coatings, chewable form, and liquid form. Often your doctor's office will have samples for you to try. If you find one that you prefer, request a prescription for that brand. Sometimes the pharmacy will oblige, but often your health insurance provider will pay for only specific brands and generic medications or vitamins.

Many patients have complained that prenatal vitamins cause nausea, especially during the first trimester when you may be feeling a bit queasy anyway. If this is happening to you, try taking the vitamin in the evening, after eating a meal. You might also consider taking the vitamins every other day. It's better than not taking any vitamins at all. The nausea should decrease as your pregnancy progresses.

6.   I'm over age thirty-five; do I need genetic testing?

If you will be thirty-five or older at the time of your delivery, your doctor will probably discuss genetic testing during your first prenatal visit. That's because studies have shown that women over the age of thirty-five have an increased chance of delivering babies with genetic abnormalities. (However, remember that the majority of these same women deliver healthy babies.)

It is important to begin the decision-making process early, because genetic testing is usually done at between 10 and 16 weeks. There is much to be done before the procedure can be performed. For example, your doctor may order an ultrasound to confirm your due date and that your baby is viable. Commonly, your doctor will refer you to a high-risk specialist to perform the actual procedure, so an appointment must be made with that physician. Finally, your health insurance provider will probably require prior authorization for this expensive and highly specialized procedure.

One of the more common genetic abnormalities that may result when the mother is over age thirty-five is Down syndrome. Down syndrome is usually compatible with life. However, children with Down syndrome are mentally challenged and also have physical defects. Besides Down syndrome, other rare genetic abnormalities may occur that cause severe problems or may be fatal.

Various charts are available that calculate the odds of these chromosomal abnormalities occurring. Talk with your doctor or with a high-risk specialist to get their opinion about your specific case. From the chart, you can see that at maternal age forty, there is still a good chance that the baby will be normal. If the chances are 1 in 65 that the fetus has some type of abnormal chromosome, then 64 times out of 65, the chromosomes should be normal.

Many women ask why the age of thirty-five has been chosen as the threshold for genetic testing. The reason is that studies show that at age thirty-five, the chance of delivering a baby with a genetic abnormality equals the chance of miscarrying as a result of the genetic testing

Baby in Womb

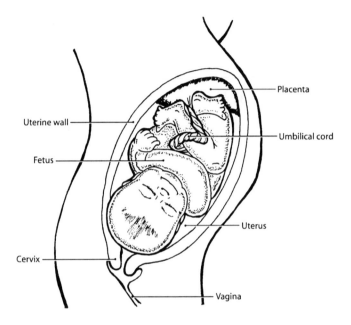

Placenta

Uterine wall

Umbilical cord

Fetus

Uterus

Cervix

Vagina

procedure itself. After age thirty-five, the chances that a woman will deliver a genetically abnormal baby are higher than the chances that she will suffer a miscarriage from procedural complications. Naturally, miscarriage and complication rates vary. Having the procedure done by an experienced and trained professional who specializes in genetic testing reduces your chance of miscarriage or postprocedural complications.

This is why your own doctor may refer you to a high-risk specialist to perform the genetic testing procedure. If you will be thirty-five or older at the time of delivery, it is important that you are informed about your options regarding genetic testing. You may elect to do nothing and go with the odds that the baby will be normal. Or you may decide to pursue genetic testing to evaluate the genetic status of the baby. It is your doctor's role to educate you and to give you options. Once you have this knowledge and the tools for understanding, the decision is yours.

Chromosomal Abnormalities by Maternal Age

Maternal Age at Delivery	Down Syndrome	All Chromosomal Abnormalities
20	1 in 1667	1 in 526
25	1 in 1250	1 in 476
30	1 in 952	1 in 384
35	1 in 385	1 in 204
40	1 in 106	1 in 65
45	1 in 30	1 in 20

Source: *Obstetrics: Normal and Problem Pregnancies*, Gabbe, Niebyl, and Simpson. (Churchhill Livingstone, 1986).

There are two types of genetic testing. Both are designed to evaluate the genetic status of the unborn baby. The first is amniocentesis; the second is chorionic villus sampling.

Amniocentesis

Amniocentesis is the most common genetic testing procedure and has been performed for decades. Depending on the position of the baby and the placenta, it is typically performed at between 14 and17 weeks. Amniocentesis may be done in the doctor's office or in the hospital.

Under the guidance of an ultrasound, a long slender needle is inserted through your abdomen and uterus and into the fluid-filled sac around the fetus. A small amount of fluid is withdrawn. The procedure is not painful; there is mild discomfort, similar to a pinprick or needle injection. Anesthesia is not typically given.

Once the fluid has been withdrawn, the fetus will produce more fluid to replace what was removed. The fluid sample is sent to the lab for genetic evaluation. The results will give the genetic status and the sex of the unborn baby and are usually available in one or two weeks. In rare cases, the cells do not grow and the test must be repeated.

Chorionic Villus Sampling

Chorionic villus sampling (CVS) is a genetic testing procedure that became commonly used starting in the 1990s. Depending on the position of the placenta and the baby, CVS is typically done at about 10 to 12 weeks. The procedure may be done in the doctor's office or in the hospital.

CVS requires that you position yourself on the exam table with your feet in stirrups, as if you were having a Pap test. An ultrasound is used to determine the exact placement of the fetus and the placenta. Then a small device is placed into your vagina and the doctor uses a thin, straw-like instrument to suction out a small sample of placental tissue. Most women do not find this procedure painful—it is similar to having a Pap smear or pelvic exam. Anesthesia is not required.

Once an adequate tissue sample is obtained, it is sent to the lab for genetic evaluation. Results of the unborn baby's genetic status and sex are available in one to two weeks. In rare circumstances, the cells do not grow and the test must be repeated.

CVS does not screen for open neural tube birth defects. If a CVS procedure is done, you may elect to have a specialized blood test (using blood from your arm) done at 16 to 18 weeks that will check for this particular problem.

It is difficult to compare the miscarriage rates resulting from the two procedures because CVS is performed considerably earlier in pregnancy, when more miscarriages occur naturally on their own. Thus, it is impossible to determine whether miscarriage would have occurred by itself or was due to the CVS procedure.

Comparison of Genetic Testing Procedures

	Amniocentesis	CVS
Timing of procedure	14-17 weeks	10-12 weeks
Tissue sample for genetic evaluation	Obtained from fluid sac around the fetus via abdomen with a slender needle	Obtained from the placenta via vagina with a straw-like suction device
Miscarriage risk	Probably lower than CVS	Probably higher than amniocentesis
Detection of other abnormalities	Screens for open neural tube birth defects	Does not screen for open neural tube birth defects
Other known complications	None	Chance of limb abnormalities (very rare)

7. When do I choose a hospital and the type of birth I'll have?

During the first prenatal visit, you may be asked to make certain decisions regarding hospitalization and type of birth. Initially, a doctor will assume you expect to eventually have a normal vaginal delivery. However, if you have had a previous C-section, you and your doctor will need to explore the best options for you.

Hospital Choice for Delivery

Your health insurance coverage and your choice of a doctor will narrow your hospital selection considerably. Assuming that you still have a choice to make, here are some considerations when selecting a hospital for your delivery.

- The location of the hospital should be no more than thirty minutes from your home or work.
- The hospital should have twenty-four-hour anesthesia coverage for emergency C-sections and also for labor pain management.
- The hospital should have an intensive care unit for newborns in case specialized medical attention is needed.

There are advantages and disadvantages to using a university or "teaching" hospital. Although at this type of hospital, interns and residents may be even more involved in your delivery than your own doctor is, the twenty-four-hour resident coverage allows for immediate action should an emergency arise.

If the hospital is not a teaching hospital, then you will likely receive more personalized care from your own physician. However, if an emergency occurs, you may have to wait until your physician arrives to handle the situation.

Once the hospital has been selected, you may sign up for their newsletter, prenatal classes, and hospital tours. The hospital may also send you various insurance and admitting forms to be completed prior to your admission and delivery. As your due date nears, your doctor's office will send a copy of your office chart to the hospital so the hospital staff will have your medical information available for your delivery.

Repeat C-section versus Vaginal Birth after C-section (VBAC)

If you had a C-section with your first baby, you may have the option of either scheduling a repeat C-section or electing to try a vaginal birth after C-section (VBAC). The conversation between you and your doctor about this decision will probably begin during your first prenatal visit. The conclusion you and your doctor eventually come to will be based on two major factors: 1) the type of incision made in your uterus during your first C-section, and 2) the reason you had your first C-section. More on this topic is covered in Chapter 12.

Postpartum Sterilization

If you are certain that you have completed your childbearing, this would be a good time to consider permanent sterilization. At your first prenatal visit, your doctor can provide you with brochures and detailed information on the pros and cons of the procedure. It is a good idea to begin this dialogue with your physician early in your pregnancy, for several reasons:

- Some doctors will not perform permanent sterilization procedures because of their own religious beliefs.
- Hospitals with certain religious affiliations may not permit the procedure to be done.
- Some health insurance companies require that consent forms be signed several months prior to the sterilization procedure. They want to ensure that you've thought out your options and have not made a hasty decision biased by the discomforts of advanced pregnancy or the pains of labor.

Be sure to have a conversation about this topic with your physician either at the first prenatal visit or shortly thereafter.

If you are having a planned C-section (or have an unexpected one), permanent sterilization takes only an extra five minutes and adds essentially no risks or problems to the C-section procedure. After the baby has been delivered and the uterine incision has been sewn, the two fallopian tubes are tied and cut. The procedure is also referred to as a tubal ligation, because it severs the tubes. The remainder of the surgery is identical to a C-section, with no additional complications such as pain, infection, or hormonal changes.

If you deliver your baby vaginally, the tubal ligation procedure is somewhat different. The procedure is performed either the same day or the day following delivery. When you are in the operating room, anesthesia (general or epidural) is administered; then, a one- to two-inch incision is made near your navel. Probes and grasping instruments must be used to locate the fallopian tubes. Once they are located, the tubes are tied and cut. Recent studies have shown increased complications from bleeding, infection, and anesthesia risks from this procedure. Therefore, many doctors are no longer performing this post-vaginal delivery procedure.

An excellent alternative to any type of female sterilization is male sterilization, or *vasectomy*. It is considered a much easier and less risky procedure than the traditional female tubal ligation. If discussing that option is feasible within your relationship, do consider it with your partner. Otherwise, a laparoscopic tubal procedure may be considered once your uterus has returned to normal nonpregnant size, many months from now.

8. What happens during my second prenatal visit?

Your second prenatal visit usually occurs about four weeks after the first visit. Therefore, most women are between 10 and 12 weeks along in pregnancy.

Typically, the medical assistant first calls you back into the examination area, then takes your weight and asks you to supply a urine sample. She will use a urine dipstick to check your urine sample for protein (kidney problems), sugar (diabetes), and bacteria (infection). You are then escorted to a private examination room, where the medical assistant will take your blood pressure and ask you if you are having any problems such as bleeding, cramping, nausea, or vomiting. She or he records this information on your chart and gives it to your physician.

Your physician joins you in the examination room and reviews the information with you. He or she will ask how you are feeling and whether you have special concerns or problems. Next, the doctor will request that you recline on the exam table and arrange your clothing to expose your upper pubic area. He or she will then place a conducting gel on your skin just above the pubic area, followed by the Doptone device. The Doptone is a small handheld device that uses ultrasound waves to listen to the fetal heartbeat. Because the baby is still quite small, a minute or two may elapse before the fetal heartbeat is located.

Many women bring along a spouse, partner, or close friend to share this tender and emotional event. It is an incredibly touching and special moment when you hear your baby's heartbeat for the first time.

At the conclusion of the visit, the physician will ensure that your concerns have been addressed and will ask you to make your next appointment in about four weeks. This entire visit takes only fifteen to twenty minutes.

3

Potential Issues and Concerns

As your first trimester nears the end, you've had time to think about other issues and concerns. During this time, many women become concerned about how past pregnancy terminations or losses might influence the current pregnancy. Bleeding and pregnancy are two terms that most women do not want to associate together. At best, spotting can cause needless alarm and concern. At worst, bleeding can be associated with pregnancy loss, in the form of either miscarriage or ectopic (tubal) pregnancy. Bleeding is the most common sign of miscarriage; however, it is reassuring to know that many women who do bleed during this time are able to successfully continue their pregnancies and deliver healthy babies.

If you have suffered with morning sickness, here's a bit of refreshing news. Ten weeks is usually the peak of morning sickness. Your nausea and vomiting will soon begin to dissipate.

Feeling tired lately? Do you have an almost uncontrollable desire to sleep? Extreme fatigue is especially common during the end of the first trimester. Understand that this is normal, and there is nothing wrong with you. It's all a part of the countdown to baby!

1. If I've had an abortion in the past, will it affect my pregnancy now?

Having one prior abortion usually does not affect your ability to carry a new pregnancy. If you have had two or more abortions, you are probably fine also, but less is known about the effect multiple abortions have on later pregnancies. Fortunately, the cervix (the opening to the uterus) and the uterus are usually resilient organs. Typically they go back to their normal anatomy within a few months following an abortion.

However, an exception to this general rule can occur if you had a particularly traumatic abortion accompanied by puncture to your uterus or severe postsurgical infection, requiring hospitalization and treatment. In this case you might have trouble becoming pregnant due to scarring in the lining of your uterus. If you have had a uterine puncture, depending on the size and location of the puncture, you might require a C-section, although it is not likely. Discuss your particular situation with your doctor. Sometimes your physician will want to review your previous medical records.

Another exception can occur if your cervix suffered severe trauma during previous abortions. This may lead to a rare condition called an *incompetent cervix*. An incompetent cervix is one that is so weak that it can no longer support the weight of a normal pregnancy. Your doctor may be able to predict this by measuring your cervical length on ultra sound, and to treat the condition. However, sometimes it is impossible to predict until the cervix weakens and a pregnancy loss occurs.

2. What if I've had miscarriages in the past?

Having one prior miscarriage should not affect your ability to have normal pregnancies in the future. However, if you have had two or more miscarriages in a row, your doctor may want to look for a possible underlying medical problem. The chart in this section shows possible causes or problems that may contribute to multiple miscarriages. If you are experiencing any of them, you and your physician can discuss your treatment plan.

Possible Causes of Recurrent Miscarriage

Problem	Treatment
Uncontrolled diabetes	Control with diet and medication
Lupus or other autoimmune disease	Control with medication
Thyroid disease	Control with medication, sometimes surgery
Pelvic infection	Treat with antibiotics
Abnormal uterus or cervix	Evaluate for possible surgery
Tobacco, alcohol, or drug use	Stop usage
Parents' chromosomes	Consider genetic testing

Keep in mind that in many cases, no underlying cause can be found for the miscarriages.

But if you have had two or more miscarriages in a row, your doctor may recommend special monitoring or medication. Most experts agree that if you successfully reach 13 weeks with a normal-appearing fetus and heartbeat on ultrasound, you will very likely go on to have a normal term pregnancy.

3. What can I do for morning sickness?

Nausea and vomiting during the first trimester are often called morning sickness. The truth is, it can occur at any time of the day. It is very common, occurring in about 70 percent of all pregnancies. Rising levels of pregnancy hormones cause these symptoms. Typically, symptoms begin at around week 6, peak at week 10, then subside by about week 14. Most cases of morning sickness are not harmful to you and will not hurt the fetus. Here are some ways to cope with the nausea and vomiting:

- Drink or eat clear fluids such as frozen juice bars, Popsicles,
- Jell-O, or ice
- Eat bland crackers, dry toast
- Eat the BRATT diet: bananas, rice, applesauce, toast, tea
- Eat five or six small meals each day
- Drink liquids thirty to forty-five minutes after eating solid foods
- Take prenatal vitamin with meal
- Avoid bothersome smells and odors
- Get plenty of fresh, cool air
- Sit up or stand up slowly
- Try over-the-counter medications: sea bands, vitamin B-6
- Ask your doctor for Rx medications

Your symptoms will usually go away as your first trimester comes to a close. In rare cases, morning sickness can be persistent and severe, leading to weight loss and dehydration. Here are signals for alarm that require a phone call to your physician:

- vomiting any fluid for more than one day
- losing weight
- urinating only a small amount that is dark in color
- feeling excessive thirst
- racing or pounding heart
- feeling dizzy or faint
- vomiting blood

In such cases, intravenous (IV) hydration in the hospital may be required. Sometimes, arrangements for IV home treatment with daily visits from a home health care nurse can be arranged.

Ectopic Pregnancy Symptoms and Treatment

Pregnancy Development	Symptoms	Treatment
Before 6 weeks	Few or no symptoms	Monitor pregnancy
6-8 weeks	Light or heavy bleeding Pelvic pain, one-sided	Evaluate for medical vs. surgical options
7-10 weeks	Light or heavy bleeding Severe pelvic pain, one-sided Shoulder pain Dizziness, weakness, fainting	Perform immediate surgery

4. Is it normal to feel tired and wiped out?

Yes, many pregnant women report being extremely tired, especially during the first trimester. This is due to your changing body, weight gain, and increasing levels of pregnancy hormones.

Proper rest will help. It is important to get eight hours of good sleep each night. If you are able to fit them in, naps are great, too.

Good nutrition is also important. You should consume an extra 300 calories per day during your pregnancy. Eating is sometimes difficult if you are feeling nauseated. Instead of eating three big meals, try to eat five or six small, healthy snacks or meals each day.

Some women find that exercise gives them energy. Walking is probably the best form of exercise during pregnancy. Check your heart rate to be sure that it does not exceed 150 beats per minute when you are exercising. If your heart rate is too high, so is the fetus's.

Prenatal vitamins provide the supplements that most women need. depending on your lab results from the first prenatal visit, your doctor may recommend additional minerals or vitamins. Avoid consuming more than 1,000 mg of calcium supplement tablets per day, because excess calcium can increase your chances of developing kidney or gallstones.

It is hoped that these practices will help you feel somewhat better and more energized. You should have considerably more energy as the second trimester gets under way.

5. Do I have to get rid of my cats?

No, there is no need to find new homes for your cats. The concern about cats is that they can carry a rare disease called *toxoplasmosis*. Fortunately, the incidence of toxoplasmosis in U.S. pregnancies is less than 0.1 percent. Ironically, most of those cases come from women eating raw and contaminated meat, not from contact with cats.

Nonetheless, in the rare event that you were infected with toxoplasmosis, significant damage to the fetus could occur. For that reason, it is recommended that you follow these guidelines while you are pregnant:

- avoid raw meats
- wash all fresh fruits and vegetables
- delegate someone else to clean the cat's litter box
- wear a mask over nose and mouth if you must clean the litter box

Keep in mind that toxoplasmosis is extremely rare; however, by taking these precautions, you further reduce your risk.

6. How do I know if I have an ectopic pregnancy?

Many women are surprised to learn that fertilization (the union of the sperm and egg) occurs within the fallopian tubes. As the fertilized egg continues to develop, it is supposed to move into the uterus, where it implants and grows. In the case of an ectopic pregnancy, the fertilized egg never makes it to the uterus. Instead, it tries to grow inside the tube. Rarely, it may attach itself to an ovary or other pelvic organ. An ectopic pregnancy cannot develop normally and therefore must be stopped;

otherwise, it can lead to rupture of the tube and possible severe hemor-rhage.

Ectopic pregnancy occurs at the rate of about 1 in 60 pregnancies. Sometimes, tubal pregnancies seem to happen for no obvious reason. However, we know there are risk factors that increase the chances for developing an ectopic pregnancy. Risks include:

- severe pelvic infections
- prior surgery on your fallopian tubes
- previous ectopic pregnancy
- history of infertility
- prior pelvic or abdominal surgery (scar tissue)
- endometriosis

Other potential risk factors include cigarette smoking, increasing maternal age, and whether your mother took the drug DES during her own pregnancy with you. (DES is a strong hormone that was used during the 1950s to help prevent miscarriages, but was later found to have many detrimental side effects.)

The two main symptoms of ectopic pregnancy are vaginal bleeding and one-sided pelvic pain. These symptoms may vary in intensity depending on how far the pregnancy has progressed. If your doctor suspects that you have an ectopic pregnancy, he or she will perform certain tests. The doctor will likely perform a pelvic exam, check your blood pressure and pulse, perform an ultrasound, and run blood tests to determine the level of a specific pregnancy hormone. The diagnosis may not be clear right away. Sometimes it takes a few days of obser-vation and additional testing before the diagnosis is clear.

Once the diagnosis of ectopic pregnancy has been made, treatment is largely based on how far along your pregnancy has progressed and what your symptoms are.

Early (before 6 weeks) ectopic pregnancies are difficult to diagnose due to lack of symptoms. The most common time to diagnose an ectopic pregnancy is at 6 to 8 weeks. That's when bleeding and pelvic pain are most likely to present themselves. Your doctor will evaluate your situation and discuss treatment options with you.

Sometimes a special medication may be used to dissolve the pregnancy. The drug most commonly used is methotrexate. It is more commonly used as a chemotherapy medication to treat cancer patients. If successful, this method allows the woman to keep her tube and she avoids surgery. If it is not successful, surgery may eventually be required.

If your pregnancy is farther along or if the tube has ruptured, surgery is the definitive way to treat the ectopic pregnancy. Sometimes the surgery can be accomplished through a small incision with the laparoscope. The laparoscope is a thin, telescope-like device with light that is inserted through a small opening in your abdomen. At other times, especially if significant blood loss has occurred, a larger incision and a hospital stay may be required. In either case, some or all of the tube may be removed. If the entire tube is removed, the woman must rely on the remaining tube for future pregnancies.

Whatever method is used to end the pregnancy, your blood should be checked several times during the next two to three weeks to ensure that the pregnancy hormone continues to decrease.

7.   Is vaginal bleeding normal during the first trimester?

No. And it can be frightening if it does occur. However, a small amount of bleeding (a teaspoon or so) may not indicate anything worrisome at all. For example, implantation bleeding may occur as the embryo implants into your uterine wall, usually at about 7 weeks. In addition, many women experience spotting after sex or heavy lifting because, during pregnancy, the cervix contains additional blood vessels. The majority of women who have vaginal bleeding during the first trimester continue their pregnancies and deliver healthy babies.

The main concern about early pregnancy bleeding is miscarriage. Bleeding is the most common sign of miscarriage. Report any vaginal bleeding you are experiencing to your doctor, so he or she can evaluate your pregnancy.

8.   How do I know if I'm miscarrying and what should I do?

As mentioned earlier, bleeding is the most common sign of miscarriage. You may be having a miscarriage if you experience significant bleeding (more than one-half cup), often accompanied by cramping. Sometimes you may pass large blood clots (golf-ball size) or fetal tissue.

Frustrating as it sounds, usually nothing can be done to stop a miscarriage from happening. Most people believe that miscarriage is the body's way of dealing with a fetus that is probably abnormal. Miscarriages occur in 15 percent of all pregnancies. They are sad events and many women blame themselves or search to find a reason for the miscarriage. Rarely can an answer be found. For example, work, exercise, sex, or most falls do not cause miscarriage. Physical conditions such as fright, stress, or morning sickness also do not contribute to miscarriage.

Most miscarriages seem to happen by chance and are not likely to happen again with future pregnancies. More than 50 percent of miscarriages are due to problems with the chromosomes of the fetus. These chromosomal problems occur randomly. When the egg and sperm combine, thousands of steps must be accomplished to form a normal fetus. If a mistake occurs with the number of chromosomes or the structure of a chromosome, miscarriage may occur. That's why most people believe that miscarriage is nature's way of taking care of a fetus that was not developing normally and may not have been able to survive.

After your doctor is notified that you are bleeding heavily, he or she will want to examine you and possibly order an ultrasound or special blood tests. Even after the initial test results are available, it may not be immediately clear whether or not you are miscarrying. Therefore, your doctor may need to monitor your symptoms and repeat some tests over the next few days until the diagnosis becomes clear.

If the diagnosis of miscarriage is made, talk with your doctor about your options. Some women prefer to schedule a *dilation and curettage* (D & C) procedure. The D & C is a surgical procedure whereby the doctor removes the pregnancy from your uterus. This is usually performed in a surgical facility while you are heavily sedated. Other women prefer to avoid surgery and choose to pass the fetus and tissue naturally, on their own. In this case, your doctor may prescribe a medicine that will cause cramping and assist tissue passage. If you choose this option, contact your doctor if your bleeding is extremely heavy (soaking a pad over a one- or two-hour period) or if you are experiencing severe pain.

If you have two or more miscarriages in a row, your doctor may want to evaluate you to determine whether a possible underlying problem is the cause.

Part II
Second Trimester

4

Lifestyle and Habits

You've reached the second trimester! Hopefully your concerns from early pregnancy have dissipated and you are feeling better both mentally and physically. As you get on with your daily life, you may have many questions about lifestyle habits and routines. For example, what types of activities are safe during pregnancy and what activities might not be such a good idea? You may have questions about over-the-counter medications, diet modifications, bathing and swimming, and sexual activity. These are good questions to ask, and all are questions commonly asked by mothers-to-be.

1. What over-the-counter medicines can I safely take?

Most doctors recommend avoiding all medications during the first trimester, if possible. That's because the fetus is developing major organ systems during that time period. However, during the second and third trimesters, some over-the-counter (OTC) medications may be considered. (See table.)

The table below lists medications that you should avoid while you are pregnant. Do not take these medications unless your doctor has specifically given you approval.

Commonly Recommended OTC Medications

Problem	Medications*
Antihistamines	Benadryl, NasalCrom, Unisom
Decongestants	Actifed, Sudafed
Antinauseant	Vitamin B-6, Dramamine, Unisom, Emetrol
Sore throat	Chloraseptic, Sucrets, Cepacol
Cough	Robitussin or Triaminic
Constipation	Surfak, Colace, Pericolace, Metamucil, Fiberall
Diarrhea	Imodium, Kaopectate
Heartburn or indigestion	Maalox, Mylanta, Tums, Rolaids, Zantac, Tagamet
Pain or headache	Tylenol (acetaminophen) or Tylenol Extra Strength
Yeast infection	Monistat (apply only halfway in vagina)

*To be absolutely certain the medication is safe for you and your pregnancy, ask your doctor.

Under certain circumstances, your doctor may approve the use of some of the medications shown in the second chart. What your doctor says about your particular situation takes precedence over the information given here.

OTC Medications to Avoid

Medications to Avoid	Reason to Avoid
Motrin, Advil, Ibuprofen, Naproxen, Aleve, all NSAIDs	Could reduce the amniotic fluid around the baby, damage baby's kidney function
Aspirin, Excedrin, Alka-Seltzer, Pepto-Bismol, other aspirin medications	May cause increased bleeding in mother or baby due to aspirin content
NyQuil or other medicines with high alcohol content	Could hurt baby due to alcohol content

2.   How can I get calcium into my diet if I don't like milk?

You're right to be concerned about having a sufficient amount of calcium in your diet, particularly now that you're pregnant. Pregnant women require about 1,200 milligrams of calcium every day (that's about the amount in four eight-ounce glasses of milk). Calcium helps to build strong bones and teeth in the unborn baby.

Milk is a great source of calcium, but if you don't like milk, you do have other choices. Yogurt, cheese, pudding, ice cream, cottage cheese, salmon, and spinach are all good sources of calcium. If these do not appeal to you, consider taking calcium supplements. First, check your prenatal vitamin to see how much calcium it contains. Then ask your doctor or dietitian about adding a calcium supplement. Many women choose Tums because they are a good calcium source and also help with indigestion.

3.   Can I consume caffeine while I'm pregnant?

Most experts agree that caffeine in moderation (less than 300 milligrams, or three cups per day) seems to present little if any risk to the fetus. However, high doses of caffeine have been linked to miscarriage, low birth weight, and premature birth. Here is a guide to common drinks and their caffeine doses.

It is best to avoid caffeine altogether, but consuming it in low to moderate levels should have little or no influence on the fetus.

Caffeine Levels

Food or Beverage	Caffeine in mg.
Average cup of coffee	100
Average cup of tea	50
Average can of cola	40
One ounce semisweet square baking chocolate	25

4. How much weight should I be gaining?

Just about every woman is concerned about weight gain during pregnancy. Total weight gain for a healthy pregnancy is approximately thirty pounds. If you were overweight before pregnancy, you may gain a little less. If you were underweight before pregnancy, you may gain a little more. Much of pregnancy weight gain is retained water and fluids.

Also consider the weight of the placenta, the amniotic fluid, and of course the fetus. The average term baby weighs 7 ½ pounds.

Pregnancy is not the time to try low-calorie or fad diets. Your unborn baby needs nutrients and you are the only source. It is important to eat a sensible and well-balanced diet.

Pregnant women often gain up to five pounds during early pregnancy. Many women gain another ten pounds in the second trimester and often more than ten pounds in the third trimester.

Weight gain in excess of about thirty-five pounds places you at higher risk of developing diabetes and high blood pressure during pregnancy. Talk with your doctor if you are concerned about weight gain.

5. Is it safe for me to bathe and swim?

Water can be very relaxing and refreshing. This is especially true during pregnancy. Long showers, baths, and swimming pool activities can be very comforting. To be safe, you should always be sure that the water temperature is 100 degrees or below. Beware of hot tubs and Jacuzzis because the water temperature is often set between 110 and 120 degrees, too high for a pregnant woman. Those very high temperatures can cause harm to the fetus, especially during early pregnancy.

Lakes and oceans are generally considered safe, but use good judgment if there are rough surges or high waves that could cause you injury. Remember, your balance may not be as good as it was prior to pregnancy.

Finally, if your bag of water has ruptured, many doctors recommend that you not submerge in any body of water. Why is this important to know? Some women, after their water breaks, wish to bathe prior to going to the hospital. A shower is fine, but avoid a bath since the risk of infection is higher if you are submerged in a tub. Ask your own doctor for his or her particular recommendation.

6. Is it okay to have sex during pregnancy?

Yes, having sex is usually fine unless your doctor has specifically advised against it. The fetus is protected by the fetal sac, your closed cervix, and a thick mucus plug that builds up over your cervix when you are pregnant. However, you may find that sex is a little uncomfortable during pregnancy. Sometimes, changing positions can help.

Many women report not having much interest in sex while they are pregnant. This may be due to their changing bodies, pregnancy hormones, fatigue, and generalized discomfort, These feelings are perfectly normal.

It is fairly common to have a scant amount of bleeding (less than a teaspoon) after sex. This occurs because your cervix has more blood vessels when you are pregnant. However, if bleeding seems excessive or if you are worried, contact your doctor.

If you have the following high-risk conditions, your doctor may recommend that you abstain from sex:

- threatened miscarriage
- premature labor or bleeding
- prior pregnancy loss
- placenta previa (placenta covering the cervix increases risk of
- bleeding)
- ruptured bag of water

7. Can I color or chemically treat my hair during pregnancy?

Yes, you may color, highlight, or chemically treat your hair during pregnancy. No proven data suggest that hairstyling products are harmful to the fetus.

However, many women have reported that these chemical products do not work as well on their hair when they are pregnant. Women are frequently disappointed when the color or results do not meet their expectations.

Pregnancy hormones are the most likely reason for these results. Also, because of these hormonal changes, many women lose a fair amount of their hair during pregnancy. Be reassured that your hair should return to normal within six months after delivery.

8. Are bleeding gums and occasional nosebleeds normal?

By the time you begin your second trimester, pregnancy has begun to cause an overall increase in your blood volume and also a change in your blood clotting factors. For these reasons, it is now more common for your gums to bleed when you brush your teeth and to experience more nosebleeds than you had before you became pregnant.

To reduce the bleeding when you brush your teeth, try brushing with a soft-bristled brush. However, as long as the bleeding does not seem excessive, it is probably not a concern. Talk with your doctor if you are worried about it.

The treatment for nosebleeds is the same whether you are pregnant or not. Tilt your head back; apply pressure with a cold compress. When the bleeding stops, you may apply petroleum jelly or another thick moisturizer to your nostrils, and sleep with a humidifier in your bedroom. Saline nose drops can be comforting. The moisture may help prevent future nosebleeds. In cases of excessive bleeding, your doctor may refer you to an ear, nose, and throat specialist to have your nasal blood vessels cauterized.

If your bleeding seems excessive, be sure to discuss it with your physician. Normally, your doctor will check your blood for anemia at your first prenatal visit and again at the beginning of the third trimester. If necessary, your doctor may recommend you take iron or other supplements.

9. Can I have dental work done while I'm pregnant?

It's best to wait until after you deliver to have cosmetic and routine cleaning or checkup dental work done. That's because the mouth is full of bacteria and whenever the dentist works on your teeth and gums or conducts a routine cleaning, large volumes of bacteria are released into your body. These could potentially cause harm to the baby. It's not worth taking that risk for cosmetic dentistry or a routine cleaning or checkup that could easily be done after the delivery.

On the other hand, if you have a tooth abscess or oral infection, then treatment may become necessary. Antibiotics may be given as a preventative measure and may help to protect the baby. Likewise, if you are having tooth pain, see your dentist for evaluation and treatment. Dental X-rays should not be taken during the first trimester. X-rays may be taken later in pregnancy (with a lead-shielded apron covering your abdomen) if medically necessary.

Dentists are usually knowledgeable about which medications you can and cannot receive during pregnancy. If they are not, they typically contact your OB/GYN physician.

10. Why am I having skin problems such as acne, rash, moles, and discoloration?

The increase in pregnancy hormones may cause your skin to be more oily and sensitive, much like it was when you were a teenager. Acne is very common during pregnancy. To treat it, it's fine to use over-the-counter creams containing benzoyl peroxide, a chemical commonly found in acne medication. However, avoid acne treatments containing Retin-A; this topical skin cream contains high levels of vitamin A that could damage your skin, which is very sensitive now. Also, it's possible that the absorption of the vitamin A into the mother's body could harm the fetus.

Some women develop an itchy, red rash associated with pregnancy. The medical term for this rash is *pruritic urticarial papules* and *plaques of pregnancy*, more commonly known as PUPPs. Your body metabolizing certain pregnancy hormones causes PUPPs. It is not dangerous to you or your baby but can be very uncomfortable. Fortunately, your doctor can prescribe medications to make you more comfortable. Because it is directly related to pregnancy hormones, the ultimate treatment for PUPPs is delivery of the baby.

Pregnancy hormones can also lead to skin discoloration. You may notice that existing moles become larger and darker, or you may develop new moles. Also, the skin around your nipples, your naval, and the midline in your lower abdomen will probably all turn darker compared to the surrounding skin color. Within a few months after your delivery, these skin changes will diminish and your skin should return to normal.

5

Special Blood Testing, Fetal Movement, and Ultrasounds

During your second trimester, you will continue to have routine monthly visits with your health care provider. You'll also have some additional health choices to make for you and your baby. For example, during the first part of your second trimester, you will be asked if you wish to take tests designed to help detect birth defects or problems with the pregnancy. This chapter will help you understand the pros and cons of such tests.

On a more exciting note, this is also the time when you usually get your first glimpse of the baby through the use of ultrasound. You'll be truly amazed to see that growing child in your belly!

1. Should I take a blood test to check for fetal abnormalities?

You will be asked at about 15 to 18 weeks whether you wish to take the alpha feto-protein plus (AFP plus) blood test. The test is designed to check for abnormalities in the unborn baby, such as open neural tube defects (skin does not properly cover the brain or spine) and several other genetic abnormalities including Down syndrome. The test is most accurate when performed during this time period.

For this simple procedure, blood is drawn from your arm and sent to the lab. The fetus is not injured in any way. The lab results take about one week.

A normal result is reassuring, and no further testing is required. Abnormal results do not always mean that something is wrong with the baby, but additional testing is recommended. Your doctor may order an ultrasound or recommend an amniocentesis to provide further information.

Many women complain about the AFP plus test. They report that they worry needlessly about an initially abnormal result that proves to be false in subsequent testing. Keep in mind that this test cannot specifically tell whether your baby has a problem. It can only predict which pregnancies may have an increased risk for certain problems. Most women with abnormal results deliver perfectly normal babies. For example, of the results showing a pregnancy with increased risk of Down syndrome, only about 2 percent of the babies born actually have the genetic abnormality.

The decision to undergo the AFP plus test is yours. It depends on what you would do with the test result information. If you would not have an abortion under any circumstances, then perhaps you should decline the test, because the results may cause you undue worry. On the other hand, if you want to have as much information as possible and want all your options available, then you should consider taking the test.

2. When should I feel the baby move?

Most women begin to feel the baby move at between 16 and 20 weeks. If this is your first baby, it may be closer to 20 weeks. Most women report that the movement starts out much like a fluttering or "butterflies in the lower abdomen" type of feeling. Sometimes it happens quickly and by the time you notice the feeling, it's gone.

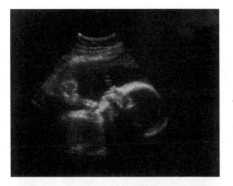

Traditional Ultrasound

Traditional, two-dimension, ultrasounds play an important role in prenatal care. Physicians use the ultrasound to check the health of the growing fetus and the mother.

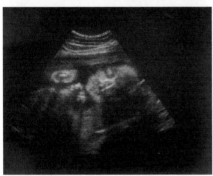

Two-dimensional ultra sounds are usually ordered between 18 and 20 weeks. The two-dimension photos show a "slice" of the fetus.

Don't expect to feel constant or regular movement until sometime during the third trimester. For right now, just know that you will occasionally feel little flutters and movements that over time will become considerably stronger and more regular.

3.   When do I get an ultrasound and what is involved?

What an exciting prospect, seeing an image of your baby for the first time! One of the highlights of your pregnancy, the ultrasound prenatal visit is usually scheduled at between 18 and 22 weeks of pregnancy. (Because insurance companies typically reimburse for only one or two ultrasounds, the ultrasound is scheduled to maximize seeing the anatomy. Therefore, the optimum time to schedule the ultrasound is during this time period.)

The ultrasound is usually performed at your doctor's office. You might see your doctor during this visit, but the ultrasound is performed by an ultrasound technician who is highly skilled at viewing the fetus by ultrasound.

Typically, you are asked to recline on the exam table, lights are dimmed, and gel and transducer are applied to your belly. The transducer uses ultrasonic waves to project an image of your baby onto a television-like monitor. There is no pain for either you or the baby. The whole procedure takes about thirty minutes.

An ultrasound provides a wealth of information. The fetal anatomy and development of major organ systems can be studied. Often the sex of the baby can be determined. Measurements of the baby's head, abdomen, and thigh are used to calculate estimated weight. The ultrasound can provide other valuable information, such as:

- number of fetuses
- position of fetus
- age and growth of fetus
- some birth defects
- location of placenta
- amount of amniotic fluid
- blood flow between fetus and placenta

In addition to the standard ultrasound done at between 18 and 20 weeks, it may be medically necessary for your doctor to order additional ultrasounds.

Reasons for Additional Ultrasounds

Symptoms or Issues	Purpose
Bleeding or cramping in early pregnancy	Rule out miscarriage or ectopic pregnancy
Unknown last menstrual period	Establish due date
High-risk factor: twins, placenta previa, diabetes	Closely monitor development
Baby not growing appropriately	Monitor growth of fetus
Possible problem with anatomy	Check for resolution or improvement
Unsure of fetal position near the due date	Check position of fetus before labor begins

Many women say that once they've seen the baby on ultrasound, they feel an increased sense of love and connection. You can expect this bond to grow stronger as you proceed through your pregnancy.

4. What are three-dimensional ultrasounds?

The relatively new technology for ultrasound is the three-dimensional model. The quality of the pictures is outstanding; you can get a clear look at your unborn baby. The image you see resembles an actual photograph. It's quite different from traditional ultrasound images that sometimes make the fetus look like an alien or skeleton, and leave many people disappointed.

However, at this time, the routine ultrasound ordered by your doctor will not be three-dimensional. In fact, 3-D ultrasounds are not considered medically diagnostic in pregnancy. That means that they don't do measurements or check anatomy, and a physician does not review their images. Instead, they are considered entertainment and fun.

Because of this, most insurance companies will not pay for this service. Facilities that perform the three-dimensional ultrasound include various doctors' offices (perhaps yours) and radiology groups. These

3-D Ultrasound

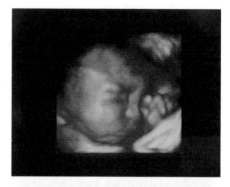

The sophisticated three-dimensional sonograms show the fetus much more clearly than the traditional two-dimensional ultrasound photos.

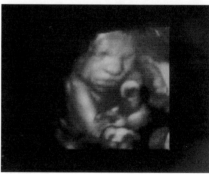

The three-dimensional ultrasounds may be performed between 26 and 30 weeks; however, they are not routinely ordered for medical purposes.

places usually insist that you have a traditional ultrasound at your own doctor's office first. If an abnormality or birth defect is noted, your own doctor will address it with you.

Like any ultrasound, the quality of the image varies depending on the size of the baby and how the baby is positioned. The optimum time to have a three-dimensional ultrasound is between 26 and 30 weeks.

Some three-dimensional ultrasounds offer various options and packages, much like a photographer's studio. Choices include still photos, video, black-and-white or color, captions, and music. The standard 15-minute, three-dimensional ultrasound costs about $150. Upgrades and options are extra, of course.

Special Blood Testing, Fetal Movement, and Ultrasounds

In a few areas of the country, a small number of high-risk specialists have begun to use this new technology for improved diagnosis of birth defects. In this situation, the patient's regular OB/GYN physician will have already detected a potential problem or birth defect during the traditional ultrasound. He or she then refers the patient to the high-risk specialist, who will take a better look at the area in question with the three-dimensional ultrasound. In this case, the 3-D ultrasound aids in pinpointing the diagnosis and is a helpful tool in explaining the problem to the patient. This is a relatively new use of this technology and it is uncertain whether or not insurance companies will pay under these circumstances. At the present time, this technique is being used by only a handful of high-risk centers in the United States.

6

Preparing for Baby

The countdown continues! In a few short months, you'll be a mother. Still, there is much to think about, and much to plan. Now is the perfect time to start preparing for the baby's arrival by purchasing items for baby, signing up for prenatal classes, considering a birth plan, and selecting a pediatrician.

You can feel more secure about the pregnancy at this point because the chances of miscarriage or other such problems are greatly reduced. If you chose to have any type of special blood or genetic testing, you should have the results by now. And, you've already seen your baby on ultrasound. Most of all, you are probably eager to make preparations for the baby's arrival because your belly is pushing outward and you are beginning to feel new life moving inside you! Chances are that most of your family and friends are aware of your exciting news and are eager to help you get started.

1.   What do I need to buy before the baby arrives?

Items for the baby may be purchased at any time during your pregnancy, but many women seem to enjoy starting to shop during the second trimester. That's because the uncertainties of early pregnancy are gone and the movement of the baby growing inside makes the entire experience seem very real and imminent.

Items Needed for Baby

Clothing	Gear or Equipment	Feeding	Nursery	Toys
Snap-up bodysuits	Car seat	Breast pump	Crib and mattress	Musical chimes
T-shirts, bibs	Carrier, pack	Bottles	Bassinet	Soft cloth toys
Socks, booties	Stroller	Nipple lotion	Changing table	Rattles
Hat	Baby bathtub	Breast pads	Monitor	Playmat
Homecoming outfit	Diapers, pail	Formula	Rocking chair	Arches and gym
Clothing related to climate	Baby blankets	Pacifiers	Night-light	Baby mirror

The most important item to purchase is an infant car seat. Be sure to take it to the hospital with you when you deliver your baby. Most hospitals won't allow you to drive the baby home without one. And don't forget to take your baby's homecoming outfit to the hospital!

Not all mothers will need all of these items. For example, if you are planning to breast-feed, you may want to buy or rent a breast pump and purchase breast pads to protect your clothing. Having nipple oil or lotion is also helpful. But if you plan to bottle-feed, then only bottles and formula are necessary. Similarly, some women prefer to keep the baby in a bassinet near their own bed for the first few months. If you feel this way, you will not need a crib and mattress until the baby is a little older.

2. Can I paint the walls in the nursery?

As long as the room is well ventilated, painting the walls should be fine, at least technically. However, do be careful if you are using a ladder. Remember, your center of balance is different now and your risk of falling has increased. Even though there is no known harm to the fetus, most physicians recommend that you relax and have someone else paint the walls.

3. Should I sign up for prenatal classes?

Yes! Prenatal classes are very important. They help you know what to expect as your body goes through the changes of pregnancy and they prepare you emotionally for the upcoming delivery and challenges of motherhood. Often, the other women in the classes have the same problems and concerns that you do. Usually begun in the seventh month of pregnancy, prenatal classes can provide a great support system.

The instructor is usually a nurse who has had specialized training in childbirth education. In addition to your childbirth educator, many prenatal classes have guest speakers. These may include a labor nurse, an anesthesiologist, a nursery nurse, and a pediatrician. It's helpful to hear their perspectives and thoughts on pregnancy and childbirth.

Prenatal classes that are offered through the hospital usually provide a tour of the maternity birthing center. You'll become familiar with the labor and delivery department and know where to go and what to expect on your big day. Hopefully, that will relieve a lot of your concerns about the birthing process.

Specialized prenatal classes are sometimes offered. For example, some hospitals or clinics offer classes for early pregnancy. They focus on the first trimester and its issues and concerns. Other classes that may be available include programs just for dads or just for siblings, and classes on baby CPR and breast-feeding.

Check with your insurance company to determine if they offer special prenatal programs. Some health insurance companies will give you special incentives and baby supplies if you meet their requirements for prenatal care visits and patient education.

4.   What is a written birth plan and should I prepare one?

A written birth plan outlines your preferences relating to the details of your upcoming birthing process. This plan specifies your wishes regarding pain management, delivery room environment, and handling of your newborn. Typically, you write it with input from your partner. The plan is subsequently discussed with and approved by your physician and then placed in your medical record. It will be made available to the medical staff in the labor and delivery unit for their review when you are admitted to deliver your baby.

There are both advantages and disadvantages to having a written birth plan.

Advantages

- May provide you with a sense of control and security to have a generalized plan
- May provide you with a better understanding of the labor and delivery process
- Becomes part of your medical record and expresses your wishes and desires to the entire medical staff

Disadvantages

- May set up unrealistic goals and expectations, resulting in disappointment or postpartum depression
- May not be revised when labor is longer or more painful than you expected
- May not provide the flexibility to deal with unexpected complications that frequently arise during the birthing process

Ask your doctor if he or she thinks a written birth plan is best for your situation. Most doctors seem to prefer good communication and rapport with each patient during those eight or nine months of prenatal visits over a written directive noted in the patient's chart. That's why it is so important for you and your doctor to discuss your expectations, wishes, and concerns during your entire pregnancy. The most important thing you can do is maintain open and honest communication with your doctor.

Whether or not you elect to have a written birth plan, please be open-minded and flexible about your birthing process. The best-laid plans can (and often do) go awry. Chances are good that your birthing experience may not go exactly as you had mapped out. If you are educated about your options and trust your doctor, you can go with the flow and not be disappointed if you veer off your planned course. After all, the main goal is always a healthy mother and baby.

5. How and when do I select a pediatrician for my baby?

Although pediatricians do not deliver babies, they are specialists in caring for infants and children. You will need to select a pediatrician before your baby is born. This doctor must examine your newborn and confirm that he or she is in general good health before you may take your baby home.

As with searching for any other physician, word of mouth is best. Ask your friends, coworkers, neighbors, nurses, and your OB/GYN doctor for recommendations. You may consider interviewing several pediatricians to see whom you prefer. The doctor you choose should meet the following criteria:

- Is board-certified
- Has privileges at your delivering hospital
- Examines or evaluates baby after delivery
- Has both a sick and well entrance to office
- Has a nurse available to answer phone calls during office hours
- Is easy to schedule an appointment with
- Has after-hours 24/7 emergency availability
- Has a partner or nurse practitioner available as backup
- Is on your insurance list

In addition to those considerations, you may also wish to ask the pediatrician other questions to ensure you share similar philosophies on important baby issues. Possible questions might include:

- How do you feel about breast-feeding versus bottle-feeding?
- Do you recommend circumcision?
- What do you think about vaccinations and well-baby checkups?
- What is your child-rearing philosophy?

7

Potential Problems and Premature Delivery

As you complete your second trimester, many of the concerns and worries of early pregnancy are behind you. Hopefully, you feel physically healthy and are brimming with excitement and anticipation. It's reassuring to feel the baby moving with more strength and consistency every day.

Still, if you are carrying twins or have some other risk factor for premature delivery, you probably have some concerns about your delivery. This chapter will help you to develop a better understanding of these issues and how they are managed.

1.   What if I have an incompetent cervix?

An *incompetent cervix* is a cervix that is weak and cannot support the weight of a growing pregnancy. A rare condition, an incompetent cervix continues to weaken under the pressure of the growing pregnancy until delivery occurs. The process is usually painless. Unfortunately, delivery occurs most commonly during the second trimester when the baby is extremely premature.

Diagnosis of incompetent cervix is difficult because it's not possible to examine the cervix and evaluate its strength to hold a pregnancy. However, an ultrasound may help to provide an estimate of the strength of the cervix because it can evaluate the length of the cervix. Then, if a problem is anticipated, frequent follow-up ultrasounds can be done to ensure that the cervical length remains stable. If the cervix begins to shorten, concern for weakening and incompetence is greatly increased. Causes of incompetent cervix include:

- trauma to cervix during difficult dilation or extensive cone biopsy
- lacerations from previous delivery
- congenital defects associated with uterine abnormalities
- pregnant woman's mother took DES (a hormone given to pregnant women decades ago to avoid miscarriage)
- abnormal cervical tissue (reduced collagen and strength fibers in the cervix)

If you have an incompetent cervix, your doctor may recommend a *cerclage procedure* to strengthen your cervix and prevent dilation. This procedure is usually performed at about 12 weeks, after a live fetus has been confirmed on ultrasound.

Your physician will probably perform this minor surgical procedure in an outpatient surgical center. You are given an epidural or similar anesthetic to ensure that you experience no pain or discomfort. A cerclage is essentially a tough band of suture sewn around the cervix (like a purse string) to hold the cervical tissue tightly together and better support the pregnancy. The entire procedure takes about thirty minutes. Extra monitoring of your pregnancy may then be required. Physical activity may be limited and sexual intercourse is often prohibited.

At approximately 37 weeks, the cerclage is removed by the doctor, usually in the office. Some women deliver soon thereafter. Others may not deliver for several weeks.

Unfortunately, you may not know that you have an incompetent cervix until you have already experienced a second trimester loss. However, once the diagnosis has been made, cerclage placement near the end of the first trimester of your next pregnancy will often save that pregnancy.

2.   Why is having twins a high-risk pregnancy?

If you are expecting twins, you know how exciting the idea of delivering two babies is! You also are probably aware of the special prenatal care you need. Twin births are considered high-risk because they are associated with additional medical problems and concerns.

The complication rate is higher with twins for many reasons. First, your uterus is actually made to carry only one fetus. Sometimes, when the uterus has grown to the size of a full-term single-sized baby, your body will go into labor. The uterus cannot distinguish between one full-term infant and two premature twins. Also, with twins your body has considerably more fluid and hormones. These added materials can raise your blood pressure, increase your weight gain, and even increase the likelihood of your developing diabetes during the pregnancy. The possibility that your babies will be born with birth defects also increases. In addition, twins mean not only two babies, but two placentas, two cords, and so forth. The chances of an incident occurring are increased based on the additional number of items that could interact and complicate the pregnancy. Here are some complications associated with twin pregnancies:

- premature delivery
- growth problems
- high blood pressure
- increased birth defects
- placental abruption (placenta tears away from the uterus)
- placenta previa (placenta covers the cervix)
- umbilical cord accidents
- abnormal positions and presentations
- increased chance of C-section

Despite these potential problems, twins are incredibly exciting and a wonderful blessing for you. Your doctor will monitor your twin pregnancy more closely than if you were pregnant with just one baby. You will likely have additional ultrasounds to evaluate the twins' growth and development. You may also have more office visits and pelvic exams. The risk of premature delivery is a main concern. Because of this, you may be required to limit your physical activity and refrain from having sex while pregnant. If premature labor does occur, you may be hospitalized or treated with medications in an attempt to stop labor.

3. What happens if I go into premature labor?

In your second trimester, if you experience spotting, painful contractions, or bloody mucus vaginal discharge, you could be going into premature labor. Let your doctor know if you experience any of these signs. Premature labor occurs when you have approximately six to eight contractions per hour and a change in your cervix. Sometimes, bleeding or breaking of your bag of water also occurs.

Once diagnosed, you may be treated with reduced physical activity, home bed rest, hospitalization bed rest, or medications (oral, vaginal, or intravenous). The goal is to prevent you from delivering early and possibly losing the baby. Premature labor does not necessarily have to mean premature delivery. Sometimes the doctor will recommend steroid injections. The purpose of these injections is to help develop the fetus's lungs in the case of premature delivery.

If premature delivery seems likely and your hospital does not have the facilities to provide the care your baby will need, you may be transferred to a hospital that specializes in the care of premature infants. About 10 percent of babies born in the United States are born prematurely.

Approximately half of the women who experience premature labor have no known risk factors. However, there are certain factors that make premature labor more likely:

- prior history of premature baby
- nonwhite race
- low socioeconomic status
- maternal age eighteen years or less
- maternal age forty years or more
- prepregnancy weight less than 100 pounds
- smoking
- cocaine or drug use
- congenital, abnormally-shaped uterus
- multiple fetuses

Premature infants, those born before 37 weeks and weighing under five pounds, have a higher chance of having neurological problems such as cerebral palsy, mental retardation, and seizures. Other serious problems related to breathing, hearing, vision, and digestive processes can occur. The earlier the baby is born, usually the more serious the problems are. However, new technologies and medications are advancing. At present, a handful of babies born at 22 or 23 weeks survive and do well. These numbers could change as new technologies, medical advances, and improved care for extremely premature infants become available. Now, however, 24 weeks most often marks the time when aggressive care will be given. By the time the fetus reaches 29 to 30 weeks, the survival rates are excellent—greater than 90 percent.

Part III
Third Trimester

8

Aches and Discomforts

You are now beginning the third trimester. Time is flying by! By this point you certainly feel pregnant and most likely have a good handle on your plans and preparations for the baby. Many women find that the third trimester brings numerous aches and discomforts. Most of these are due to the continued growth of the baby and the ever-increasing level of pregnancy hormones.

In the third trimester, you may not have the energy and vitality that you previously experienced. Your moods and emotions may also be more volatile. Rest assured that such symptoms are quite normal for this stage of your pregnancy. This chapter has some tips to help you feel more comfortable.

1. What can I do about indigestion, excessive gas, and constipation?

It's very common to have problems with your digestive system during pregnancy. That's because certain pregnancy hormones cause your stomach and bowel functions to slow down. Food stays in your body longer so you have more indigestion, gas, and constipation. In addition, as the fetus grows and presses on your bowels and rectal area, it becomes more uncomfortable and difficult to maintain normal bowel function. Here are some suggestions that may help you relieve digestive problems:

- Increase water and fluid consumption
- Increase the amount of fiber, fresh fruits, and vegetables in
- your diet
- Eat five to six small meals a day
- Take your prenatal vitamin with a meal
- Sit upright for one hour after eating
- Try over-the-counter stool softeners
- Try antacids: Tums, Mylanta, or Maalox

As always, speak with your doctor before taking any medications. Only your health provider knows your medical circumstances and what is best for your particular situation. Once the baby has been delivered, your digestive discomfort should quickly dissipate.

2.   What can I do about hemorrhoids?

As the fetus grows, more and more pressure is placed upon your rectal area, often causing the blood vessels around the rectum to enlarge. These enlarged blood vessels are a special type of varicose veins called hemorrhoids. They are very common and normal during pregnancy and do not pose any danger to you or your baby.

Unfortunately, hemorrhoids sometimes cause itching, pain, or bleeding. If the discomfort is severe, your doctor may write a prescription for medication; but in many cases, taking the following actions will offer the relief you need without a prescription:

- Drink plenty of water and liquids
- Eat a high-fiber diet with lots of fruits and vegetables
- Minimize standing for more than one hour at a time
- Lift no more than fifteen pounds
- Utilize sitz baths (warm solution of salt and water)
- Use a donut pillow

- Elevate hips and legs when possible
- Use over-the-counter stool softeners
- Use over-the-counter remedies: Tucks, Preparation H, Anusol

In case of excessive rectal bleeding, contact your doctor. Excessive bleeding is more than about one-quarter cup of bright red rectal bleeding. Your doctor will want to evaluate the amount of bleeding and possibly refer you to a colorectal surgeon for an outpatient procedure.

The determination to send you to a colorectal specialist depends on the size and quantity of your hemorrhoids and the amount of bleeding as evaluated by your physician. In the rare case that an outpatient surgical procedure becomes necessary, it is usually a minor surgical procedure to tie off and remove the hemorrhoids.

In all cases, after you deliver your baby, hemorrhoids will either completely disappear or reduce in size and symptoms dramatically.

3. Is it normal to leak urine when I sneeze, laugh, or cough?

Leaking a little urine at inopportune times can be attributed to a couple of factors when you are pregnant. First, pregnancy hormones cause your bladder muscles and the surrounding pelvic support musculature to relax more than usual. Second, the pregnant uterus is pressing on the bladder. This common problem often gets worse as the baby grows and puts more weight on your bladder.

Kegel exercises may help. These special exercises were developed to strengthen the muscles of the pelvic floor and prevent urinary leakage. Ask your doctor or nurse to help you get started. They can offer instructions and ensure you are doing the exercises correctly. You can check that you're doing the exercises correctly yourself by placing a finger in your vagina and squeezing around it. When you feel pressure around your finger, you are using the correct muscle. Try doing this exercise for five minutes twice a day, squeezing the muscle for a count of four and relaxing for a count of four.

If you are experiencing frequent and burning urination or blood in your urine, you should be checked for a possible urinary tract infection.

After the baby has been delivered, your bladder function should greatly improve. However, many women report that the pelvic muscles that once supplied tremendous bladder and vaginal support in their prepregnancy days are no longer as strong after delivering a baby. Give it time and continue doing Kegel exercises. If you are still concerned six months after the delivery, speak with your physician for evaluation.

4. What causes varicose veins and what can I do about them?

Pregnancy increases the amount of blood flowing through your system. In addition, the weight of your enlarging uterus reduces the circulation in your lower body. The reduced circulation is especially noticeable in your legs and ankles. It's no wonder that blood tends to accumulate in your lower legs, causing the veins to fill and bulge. This results in large, dilated veins called *varicose veins*. Occasionally, varicose veins cause your legs to ache and feel sore, especially after standing for long periods of time. Here are some things you can do to relieve the discomfort associated with varicose veins:

- Recline on either of your sides, not flat on your back
- Put your feet higher than your heart
- Consider wearing support or compression stockings
- Exercise your calves
- Massage your legs with soothing lotions

Varicose veins may be uncomfortable and unattractive, but rest assured that they pose no danger to you or your baby.

5. What is causing my nagging backaches and what can I do about them?

Unfortunately, backaches are extremely common during pregnancy. As your unborn baby grows, the expanding uterus causes a change in your balance and center of gravity. This may alter your posture and the way that you walk. Also, pregnancy hormones cause your back and abdominal muscles to relax and become weaker. In combination, these factors may result in back pain.

The good news is that you can do much to alleviate your back discomfort during pregnancy. Ask your doctor for a pamphlet, available to him or her through the American College of Obstetricians and Gynecologists, showing special exercises that can help relieve backache; then, build these exercises into your daily schedule. Following are other tips to reduce your backaches.

- Wear sensible shoes with good arch support
- Avoid standing for long periods of time
- Bend your legs to reach down; don't bend from the waist
- Avoid lifting more than fifteen pounds
- Ensure that chairs have adequate back support
- Use extra pillows in bed to get comfortable
- Utilize heat packs or cold packs
- Use Tylenol or BenGay
- Consider wearing a pelvic support belt or back brace
- Have a massage or physical therapy
- After your delivery, your backaches will diminish

6. How can I ease my discomfort enough to get a decent night's sleep?

Many pregnant women complain of not being able to sleep through the night. This disruption in sleep pattern has several sources. Hormonal changes and increased pressure on the bladder from the growing pregnant uterus make going to the bathroom a couple of times each night a necessity. This need is normal, but it still can keep you wakeful. Most pregnant women also have considerable trouble getting comfortable in bed. As your abdomen grows, it is harder to find a comfortable position, and it is more difficult to roll from side to side.

You may also suffer from heartburn or indigestion when lying down, due to acid reflux.

Follow these recommendations for a better night's sleep:

- Ensure that your last food or drink is taken more than two hours before bedtime
- Empty your bladder as much as possible before bedtime
- Use extra pillows under your head, feet, and side to get comfortable
- Consider sleeping in a comfortable recliner chair
- Practice meditation or other relaxation techniques
- Ask your doctor about over-the-counter medicine to help if needed
- Ask your doctor about prescription medication if needed

7. Am I okay even though my legs and feet are so swollen that my shoes don't fit?

There is considerably more blood and fluid in your body when you are pregnant than when you are not pregnant. As mentioned, the pregnant uterus also presses against some of your body's major blood vessels, making circulation less efficient. This is usually most noticeable in your arms, hands, feet, and legs; however, some women notice an overall puffiness.

Swelling alone is not a worrisome sign, although it can be quite uncomfortable and a nuisance when rings, watches, and shoes no longer fit properly. Some women remove rings to avoid them becoming stuck on their fingers. Many women buy larger shoes or opt for open-toed shoes if practical. Swelling may not be avoided entirely, but here are some ways to assist you in reducing it:

- Drink lots of water to flush out your system
- Add lemon and cucumber to foods as natural diuretics
- Eat fresh fruits and vegetables and low-salt foods
- Avoid standing for long periods
- Elevate your feet higher than your heart
- Lie on your left or right side, not flat on your back
- Enjoy walking or swimming
- Avoid fast food, restaurant food, canned foods, frozen foods,
- and cold cuts

Over-the-counter water pills or prescription diuretics are not recommended during pregnancy and could actually be harmful to you and the baby.

In rare cases, your swelling could be associated with a potentially dangerous condition of pregnancy called *preeclampsia.* Other names for preeclampsia are pretoxemia and pregnancy-induced hypertension. Preeclampsia is a form of high blood pressure that is associated with pregnancy and can potentially be harmful to you and your baby. Besides swelling, other symptoms of preeclampsia usually include high blood pressure, headaches, blurry vision, and protein in your urine. Your health care provider checks for these symptoms at each of your prenatal visits. However, if you notice increased swelling, headaches, or blurry vision in between your regularly scheduled appointments, you should notify your physician.

8. Why are my breasts already leaking milk?

Pregnancy hormones cause numerous breast changes. It is perfectly normal to have some leakage of either colostrum (clear fluid) or actual breast milk during your pregnancy. This leaking may occur more often if your breasts have been stimulated, for example, after sex or a warm bath. Do not squeeze or further stimulate your breasts and nipples, because that will activate more milk production. It may also cause premature contractions. Do wear a well-fitting and supportive bra.

In addition to the leakage, you also may notice your breasts enlarging and becoming more sensitive. Small raised areas around your nipples may appear. These are called *Montgomery's tubercles* and are a normal change in your breast tissue during pregnancy.

Do notify your physician if your nipple discharge is bloody or any other color besides white, beige, or clear. Also notify your doctor if you notice a mass or lump.

9.   What can I do about stretch marks?

Stretch marks cross areas on the body that are expanding during pregnancy. They usually can be seen on the abdomen but also can appear on your breasts, hips, and thighs. Some people are more likely to get stretch marks than others. Stretch marks are not directly related to the amount of weight you gain or how much your body expands during pregnancy. They are more likely linked to the type and amount of collagen fibers contained within your skin.

When stretch marks first appear they are often red and raised, and sometimes itchy. To alleviate discomfort, keep the areas moisturized and supple with a good cream or lotion. It won't prevent the stretch marks, but it will reduce the itching and make you feel better. Beware of the many products on the market that claim to prevent or rid you of stretch marks. I've not yet seen one that really works. After delivery and over many months, the stretch marks will fade and become less obvious.

10. What about traveling during pregnancy?

Traveling during pregnancy is usually considered to be safe. However, notify your doctor when you are planning to take a trip. You may have certain high-risk conditions that could influence your ability to travel. Even if there are no special circumstances, you will want to keep certain precautions in mind.

First, pregnancy causes a change in your blood's clotting properties. Sitting still for long periods of time (in a plane, train, or car) increases your chance of developing a blood clot in either of your legs. Symptoms of blood clot are calf pain, swelling, redness, and tenderness. Blood clots are particularly dangerous if part of the clot breaks off and goes to your lungs.

Another concern of prolonged sitting is developing a urinary infection. Fighting the urge to urinate or allowing the urine to build up in your bladder could contribute to a urinary infection.

You can easily solve both the blood clot and the urinary problem by walking around and going to the bathroom every couple of hours. It is also important to drink lots of water and remain well hydrated to avoid additional urinary problems.

Some airlines require a note from your health provider if you plan to travel after 32 weeks of pregnancy. Their primary concern is that you may deliver while in flight. There is no harm to you or the fetus in a normal commercial airline's pressurized cabin. However, it is not recommended that you fly in small planes that are not pressurized. The changes in atmospheric pressure could cause your membranes to rupture.

When traveling by car, be sure to wear your seat belt. It should be worn under the belly and across your lower lap. If you are involved in a car accident, you must go to the nearest hospital for evaluation. They will monitor the fetal heartbeat, check for contractions, and sometimes draw blood for testing.

When traveling, it is a good idea to bring along a copy of your prenatal medical record. If you need to visit an unfamiliar hospital or clinic, that record will provide valuable information to the medical personnel. If you plan to leave the country, you should talk with your doctor about possible health concerns. Perhaps you will need to avoid drinking the local water, or certain diseases particular to that region might require specialized medicines or vaccinations.

Most health care providers recommend that you stay close to home during your last month of pregnancy. The last few weeks are the most common time when you could go into labor or have other pregnancy complications.

9

Prenatal Visits, Medical Issues, and Infections

You are racing toward your due date! In some ways, you may wish the pace of the race would quicken—it is very common in the third trimester to feel big and uncomfortable. This is also a time when your health provider will want to watch you more closely for other health concerns that can occur during this time. That's why your prenatal visits will become more frequent. You will be closely monitored for such things as high blood pressure and signs of infection that could interfere with your upcoming delivery or cause potential harm to the baby.

Keep in mind that the clock is ticking. The countdown is on. Your delivery is not far off!

1. How often are prenatal visits scheduled during the third trimester?

Until now, your prenatal visits have probably been scheduled on a monthly basis. During your third trimester, the visits will occur more often.

The first visit of the third trimester typically occurs at about 26 to 28 weeks. This is an especially important visit because you will most likely be tested for pregnancy-related diabetes, also known as *gestational diabetes.*

Your prenatal visits that follow will occur more frequently, usually every two weeks for a while. The majority of the visits are similar to those experienced during the second trimester. You are weighed, your blood pressure is checked, and urine is evaluated. The physician will listen to the baby's heartbeat with the Doptone, as previously discussed. If your physician has not previously performed measurements of your *fundal height*, this becomes important during the third trimester.

Fundal height measurement is a way to assess the size of your uterus and subsequently gives an estimated size of the baby. The health provider uses a tape measure, starting at your pubic bone and running it straight up your abdomen to the top of your uterus. That number in centimeters should correspond closely to your week of pregnancy. In other words, your fundal height should measure about 34 centimeters at week 34 of your pregnancy. Discrepancies of more than two to three centimeters in either direction may call for evaluation by ultrasound to further assess the growth of the fetus.

During the very last month of pregnancy, prenatal visits are scheduled on a weekly basis. These visits include a pelvic exam as well as other routine checks. The pelvic exam determines the status of cervical dilation, if any. It also helps determine whether the baby is in the desired head-down position for labor. At this time, your doctor will be particularly attentive to any vaginal infections that might influence your upcoming delivery.

2. If my blood is Rh-negative, how does it affect my pregnancy?

If you have Rh-negative blood, your pregnancy will probably be completely normal, thanks to *RhoGAM*, a medication available since 1968. This medication prevents harm to the fetus when the mother's blood is Rh-negative and the baby's is Rh-positive.

To understand how RhoGAM can help your pregnancy, it is helpful to first have a basic understanding of blood types and the *Rh factor.* When you're told your blood type, you are usually given a letter first—A, B, O, or AB—followed by either a positive or a negative sign. The positive or negative sign indicates whether you have the Rh factor, a protein on the surface of your blood cells. The majority of people have the Rh factor and are called Rh-positive. About 15 percent of the population does not have the Rh factor; these individuals are called Rh-negative. Your Rh factor usually doesn't affect your health unless you need a blood transfusion or become pregnant. Rh-negative women require special attention during pregnancy.

The Rh status of a pregnant woman's baby is not known, but it is assumed that the baby's blood is Rh-positive because most people's blood is. However, if the mother is Rh-negative, there can be potential problems. If the baby's Rh-positive blood mixes with the mother's Rh-negative blood, a reaction in the mother's blood occurs. Her blood detects the baby's Rh protein, considers it foreign and harmful, and begins to build up attack antibodies against it. As more and more attack antibodies are made, the mother's blood begins to attack the baby's blood. The medical term for this process is called *Rh sensitization.* This action, known as *hemolytic anemia,* causes some of the baby's blood to be destroyed. This is extremely harmful to the baby, and in severe cases, brain damage or death may occur in the unborn baby.

In theory, mother and baby have completely separate blood systems, so their blood should not mix. However, we know that the blood does sometimes mix, for a variety of reasons:

- miscarriage
- abortion
- ectopic pregnancy
- CVS procedure
- amniocentesis
- abdominal trauma (car accidents, blows)

- abruption (separation) of the placenta
- delivery

The attack antibodies that the mother makes against the Rh factor will stay in her blood throughout her life. In many cases, the first baby will be fine because there was not enough time for mother's blood to make a large quantity of attack antibodies. However, future pregnancies will be harmed.

The good news is that Rh sensitization can almost always be prevented by giving an injection of RhoGAM. It prevents mother's blood from forming the attack antibodies. Thus, current and future pregnancies should be safe. If you have Rh-negative blood, your doctor will recommend a RhoGAM injection at 28 weeks and again after delivery. The dose at 28 weeks protects women who might become sensitized during their last trimester. After delivery, the baby's blood is tested. If the baby is Rh-positive, another RhoGAM injection is given to the mother. If the baby is Rh-negative, the dose already given at 28 weeks should cause no harm and the postdelivery dose is unnecessary.

In addition to term pregnancy, RhoGAM is also recommended to Rh-negative women after miscarriage, abortion, ectopic pregnancy, CVS procedure, amniocentesis, and abdominal trauma.

If you and the baby's father both have Rh-negative blood, then the baby will also be Rh-negative. Notify your doctor, and he or she may forego the RhoGAM injection. (Often the doctor will ask for proof of the father's Rh status.)

In the event that a woman is already Rh sensitized from a prior pregnancy, RhoGAM is of no value. The baby must be followed closely with specialized tests to watch for signs of hemolytic anemia. If the baby begins to show signs of disease, the baby may be given a transfusion while still in the mother's uterus, or may be delivered earlier than the originally planned due date, in order to receive the necessary treatment.

3. Why do you check for diabetes when there's none in my family history?

When you are pregnant, you are at increased risk for developing a special type of diabetes called gestational diabetes. In all pregnancies, a specific hormone, *human placental lactogen* (HPL), continues to increase as the pregnancy progresses. Most pregnancies handle this change without difficulty. However, in some circumstances this particular rising hormone changes the body's normal metabolism of sugar and insulin, resulting in gestational diabetes. This typically occurs around the beginning of the third trimester. It's very important to be tested for gestational diabetes because it can cause potential problems for both mother and baby. Here are some possible problems associated with gestational diabetes if the sugar-insulin metabolism is not closely monitored and treated:

- urinary tract infections
- fetal growth problems (too big, too small)
- high blood pressure, preeclampsia
- excessive amniotic fluid that can cause premature delivery
- increased C-section rate
- damage to shoulder and arms during delivery if baby is large
- birth defects
- fetal death
- respiratory distress for baby after birth

Most of these complications occur because the sugar level is extremely high or not well controlled during the course of the pregnancy.

Most health providers test all pregnant patients because it's difficult to predict who may develop gestational diabetes. However, certain risk factors are known to increase the chances. Keep in mind that you may still develop diabetes even if you have none of these known risk factors.

Risk Factors Contributing to Gestational Diabetes

- Obesity
- High blood pressure
- Native American
- Over age thirty-five
- Strong family history

The testing for gestational diabetes is usually done at about 26 to 28 weeks. You will be asked to drink a sweet beverage, given to you by your health provider or lab personnel. One hour later, your blood will be drawn and checked for glucose level. If the level is low or normal, no more tests are necessary because you do not have gestational diabetes. But if your glucose level is high, you will be asked to do additional testing. The follow-up test requires that you fast for twelve hours; that means nothing to eat or drink for the twelve hours prior to taking the test. The first blood drawn will be taken immediately after fasting. Then you will be asked to drink a larger volume of the same laboratory sugar beverage. For the next three hours, your blood will be drawn every hour to check your glucose level over time. If these levels are high, you may be diagnosed with gestational diabetes.

If the diagnosis of gestational diabetes is confirmed, you will be placed on a special diet. It is a well-balanced and sensible diet authorized by the American Diabetes Association. It limits sweets, fruits, and other foods high in sugar. You will be taught how to check your own blood sugar level. Your health care provider will also monitor these values closely. Usually diet alone can keep your glucose level in an acceptable range. However, if your glucose level is still too high, your physician may start you on insulin injections. (In some areas, pills to control blood sugar during pregnancy are beginning to be used.) Because of the diabetes, you are considered at high risk and you may have additional prenatal visits during your pregnancy. You may also have additional ultrasounds to monitor the growth and size of the baby.

If you watch your diet and monitor your glucose level closely, you and the baby should be healthy. Most diabetic women experience a normal labor and vaginal delivery. While you are in labor, your blood sugar level will be checked frequently. The fetus may also require additional monitoring. You and your baby may also be evaluated somewhat more closely than other patients for about twenty-four hours after delivery.

Many women who acquire gestational diabetes are concerned that they will have some form of diabetes forever. Fortunately, this is not the case. Gestational diabetes almost always goes away immediately after you deliver your baby. However, some studies indicate that women who develop gestational diabetes may be at increased risk for developing adult-onset diabetes later in their lifetimes.

4.   What is preeclampsia or pregnancy-induced hypertension?

Preeclampsia or pregnancy-induced hypertension is a special type of high blood pressure disease that can occur during the third trimester of pregnancy. This condition can be very dangerous to both baby and mother.

With preeclampsia, the mother's high blood pressure causes the baby to receive less blood flow to the placenta. As a result, the baby may receive less than optimal amounts of oxygen and nutrients. Under these circumstances, the baby's growth and development are poor.

Often the baby is born abnormally small and malnourished. The high blood pressure can also damage the mother's organ systems. In severe cases the mother can have damage to her kidneys, liver, brain, eyes, and heart.

To prevent these problems from occurring, the doctor will carefully monitor both the baby and the mother. The baby receives special fetal monitoring or ultrasound once or twice each week. This special testing is evaluated by the doctor to ensure that the baby is doing well. If the doctor determines there are problems with the baby's development, then plans for delivering the baby may be made. In addition, certain measures will be taken to help reduce or stabilize mother's high blood pressure. These include:

- bed rest at home or hospital
- blood pressure, urine, and blood count monitoring
- steroids to mature baby's lungs
- antiseizure medications (e.g., magnesium sulfate)
- blood pressure medications

No one knows exactly what causes preeclampsia; however, certain risk factors make it more likely.

Risk Factors for Preeclampsia

- High blood pressure before pregnancy
- Preeclampsia with prior pregnancy
- First baby
- Maternal age over forty years
- Twins or triplets
- Diabetes or kidney disease
- Family history of preeclampsia
- African American

Approximately 7 percent of all pregnant women are diagnosed with preeclampsia. Your doctor will evaluate you for the warning signs of preeclampsia at each third trimester prenatal visit. The need to evaluate you is actually one of the main reasons you have more frequent prenatal visits during the third trimester.

When evaluating you for preeclampsia, your physician looks for three main indicators:

- high blood pressure
- protein in your urine
- extreme swelling of your hands, feet, legs, or face

Other symptoms you may have are headaches, blurry vision, and pain in your right upper abdomen. Be sure to tell your doctor if you experience these symptoms.

Ultimately, delivery of the baby, either vaginally or by C-section, is the cure for preeclampsia. In severe cases, it sometimes becomes necessary to deliver the baby prematurely, so the baby can receive the oxygen and nutrients that it needs to develop properly.

5. What if I have a medical history of genital warts?

Genital warts do not usually cause problems with delivery, but on rare occasions, complications do occur. Therefore, it's important that your doctor knows, if you have ever been treated for them. Genital warts, also called *venereal warts*, are caused by the *human papilloma virus* and are spread through sexual contact. The warts are fleshy growths that may appear as small pink bumps on the lips of the vagina, inside the opening of the uterus, or between the vagina and the anus. Vaginal infections and pregnancy may cause warts to grow and spread. External genital warts are relatively easy to identify; however, those growing internally must be detected by a Pap test or a special microscope, called a colposcope.

If you have been diagnosed with genital warts prior to becoming pregnant, your doctor may want to perform another Pap test, a colposcope, and view your outside genital area during your third trimester. If all of these tests are normal, you can feel reassured that you will probably have a safe vaginal delivery.

In addition, if you have a history of genital warts on your cervix, your doctor will want to determine whether or not you had a surgical procedure for treatment. The two surgical procedures to treat this condition are *loop electrosurgical excision procedure* (LEEP) or *cold knife cone*. Both of these procedures involve removing a cone-shaped wedge of diseased cervical tissue. If you have had one of these procedures, there is a small chance that the postsurgical scar tissue may not let your cervix dilate properly while you are in labor, thereby slightly increasing your chance of C-section delivery. Of more concern is whether your cervix was substantially weakened because a large quantity of tissue was removed at the time of the procedure. This is extremely rare, but could lead to an incompetent cervix, resulting in a second trimester miscarriage. If you are unsure whether you've had such a procedure, you may want to ask your doctor to request your past medical records for review. Even if it is determined that you did have either of these surgical procedures, there is usually no concern about your pregnancy.

If you develop genital warts during the pregnancy, treatment is almost always withheld until after delivery. The required surgical procedure on the cervix would be too dangerous for the baby and would increase the likelihood of preterm birth or infection. In some cases, mild topical acid may be applied during pregnancy. However, this treatment is often futile; warts either grow back quickly or do not disappear because they are stimulated by pregnancy hormones.

Even if genital warts are present at the time of delivery, most women are able to deliver without any problems for mother or baby. On extremely rare occasions, the baby may develop tiny warts in the throat that require treatment by an ear, nose, and throat specialist.

6. What is Group B strep (GBS) bacteria and why will I be tested for it?

Group B strep (GBS) is not the kind of strep you commonly hear about with strep throat. It is another type of bacteria that can cause potential harm to a newborn baby, but causes no symptoms in the mother. About 30 percent of all women are natural carriers of this bacteria and almost none of them have problems or require treatment.

The concern with GBS bacteria occurs as the pregnant woman nears the time of delivery.

GBS bacteria can cause significant harm to the baby if the baby comes into contact with it during the labor and delivery process. This is especially true once the bag of water is broken. Approximately 2 percent of babies who are exposed to GBS bacteria become infected and develop severe illnesses. Potential problems include *septicemia* (blood infection), *pneumonia* (lung infection), *meningitis* (spinal infection), and death. Fortunately, the great majority of babies who are exposed to GBS bacteria do not develop an infection and remain healthy.

In an effort to avoid a GBS infection in the newborn, most health practitioners test for the presence of GBS bacteria in mother's genital area a few weeks before the due date. To test for GBS bacteria, the health provider places a cotton swab in the woman's vagina and also touches the swab along the rectal area. The cotton swab is then sent to the lab for culture and analysis. If GBS bacteria are found, then the pregnant woman will be given antibiotics during labor. Sometimes a urine sample from earlier prenatal visits may show the presence of GBS bacteria. If that is the case, antibiotics will also be given during labor.

Some physicians believe that certain pregnant women with high risk factors should be treated for GBS bacteria, no matter the culture results. By treating all pregnant women who test positive for GBS bacteria and also treating women with risk factors, the chances of the baby developing a GBS infection are greatly reduced.

High Risk Factors for GBS Bacteria

- Mother with fever during labor
- Premature labor
- Premature rupture of membranes
- More than eighteen hours since sac broke
- Prior baby with GBS infection

It is a good idea for you to know the results of your GBS test before you go into labor. This may not always be possible, because you might go into labor before your test results come back from the lab. However, if possible, it is in your best interest to know the test results. That way, if your doctor's office has not communicated with the hospital yet or if you go into labor after office hours, your necessary antibiotics can be started promptly. Most labor and delivery units will take your word that you are GBS positive and begin the antibiotics immediately. They will verify your test results once your doctor's office opens in the morning.

7. What if I have a medical history of genital herpes?

There is no way to test for the genital herpes virus unless you are currently having an outbreak with active lesions that can be cultured. Unless this is the case, the only way your doctor will know that you have a medical history of genital herpes is for you to tell him or her. It is extremely important to let your health provider know if you have had herpes outbreaks in the past. If you have, your health provider will want to monitor you more closely during the third trimester. That's because if the herpes virus is passed to the baby, usually at the time of delivery, the baby can become extremely sick. Possible complications for the baby include skin infections, meningitis (spinal infection), *encephalitis* (brain infection), blindness, mental retardation, and death. Fortunately, fewer than 1 percent of babies born in the United States are infected with the herpes virus.

If you have a herpes outbreak while you are pregnant, it usually will not harm the baby. However, if the outbreak has made you extremely uncomfortable, medications may be used to alleviate your symptoms during the second and third trimesters. (Most doctors prefer not to give medication during the first trimester.) If you have frequent outbreaks, many health care providers will recommend that you begin a preventive antiviral medication at about 36 weeks. The purpose is to minimize the chance of an outbreak just prior to delivery, thereby improving the chance of a safe vaginal delivery. If you do happen to have a herpes outbreak near the time of delivery, many doctors recommend delivery by C-section. A C-section reduces the chances of the fetus coming into contact with the virus by avoiding mother's birth canal.

Women who become infected with the herpes virus for the very first time when they are pregnant have a higher risk for problems. That's because the first herpes infection loads your body with the virus and your body hasn't had time to build up attack antibodies. Therefore, there is a higher chance that the virus could be passed to the baby through your bloodstream via the placenta while you are still pregnant.

Newborn babies who have been exposed to the herpes virus usually require intensive care treatment and are given antiviral drugs intravenously to minimize infection.

10

Bleeding in Late Pregnancy

As mentioned earlier, bleeding that occurs anytime during pregnancy is a concern that should be evaluated by your health provider. During your third trimester, there are two potentially dangerous bleeding conditions. Both of these potential complications involve the placenta. The odds are these complications won't be a problem for you, but it's good to understand their symptoms and how doctors handle them.

1. What is placenta previa and how is it managed?

The placenta is the tissue that forms a nourishment link between the mother and the baby. The placenta is about the size of a single-layer round cake and is attached to the inside of the uterus. The mother's blood supplies oxygen and nutrients on one side of the placenta, and the baby receives them on the other side through the placenta's attached umbilical cord. In most cases the placenta implants either near the top or along the sides of the uterine wall. However, in some cases, the placenta is located extremely low within the uterus. It may even partly or completely cover the cervix, the opening of the uterus. This abnormal position of the placenta is called *placenta previa*.

Placenta previa is likely to cause vaginal bleeding or extreme hemorrhage during the third trimester. Prior to that time, bleeding is less

Normal Placenta

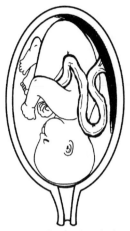

The placenta, dark-shaded area above, is the baby's lifeline. It connects to the mother's blood supply to provide oxygen and nutrients.

Complete Placenta Previa

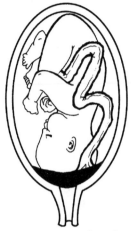

In placenta previa, the placenta implantation obstructs the opening of the cervix. The obstruction may be complete or partial.

likely because the cervix is almost always closed tightly and is filled with a large amount of protective mucus. As the third trimester continues, the cervix may dilate slightly and the protective mucus may soften and begin to dissipate. This exposes the placenta to a partially opened cervix. Activities such as sexual intercourse, exercise, and preterm labor may all stimulate the cervix and cause bleeding from the exposed placenta. Also vaginal infection may irritate the cervix and cause bleeding. Since the bleeding is due to the placenta leaking out from the cervix, the bleeding is painless. The amount of bleeding may range from mild spotting to extreme hemorrhage. Depending on the amount of blood loss, the bleeding may be life-threatening for both the baby and the mother.

Placenta previa occurs in 1 out of 175 births. The two most common contributing factors are having more than one prior pregnancy and delivery, or having prior C-sections. Placenta previa is often only diagnosed after the first episode of bleeding. An ultrasound is used to make the diagnosis.

Once placenta previa is diagnosed, certain precautions must be taken. Pelvic rest (no sex, no tampons, no douching) is usually advised in order to reduce the risk of bleeding. The mother and baby must be monitored more frequently, often by ultrasound or additional office visits. Sometimes patients are hospitalized for observation. Blood must be available for mother in the case of emergency hemorrhage requiring transfusion.

C-sections are the usual mode of delivery for patients with placenta previa. That's because during a vaginal delivery, the baby is delivered first, along with the umbilical cord, followed closely by the attached placenta. In the case of placenta previa, since the placenta is covering the cervix, the placenta would have to be delivered first. The placenta is the baby's life support system and cannot be delivered before the baby. Therefore, a C-section is almost always required for a safe delivery.

2. What is placental abruption and how is it managed?

Placental abruption refers to a condition in which the placenta either partially or completely detaches from the mother's uterine wall. The amount of detachment can vary greatly, but all abruptions must be closely evaluated. As previously mentioned, the placenta provides the link for passing oxygen and nutrients from the mother to the baby. The placenta is baby's life support system while inside the uterus. Serious consequences to both mother and baby can occur if the placenta detaches from the uterus before the baby is born. Once the placenta has detached, it cannot be reattached.

The mother will know something is wrong. Symptoms caused by the detaching placenta are intense abdominal pain and an extremely

Placental Abruption

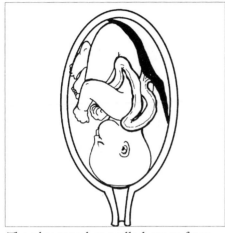

The placenta has pulled away from the wall of the uterus.

rigid abdomen that will not relax. These symptoms are almost always accompanied by bleeding from the vagina. However, on some occasions the bleeding is internal and no blood can be detected until after delivery. If these symptoms occur, the mother should call the doctor immediately and go to the hospital for further evaluation and treatment. The danger to the mother is blood loss.

For the baby, the detaching placenta reduces the amount of oxygen and nutrients being received. Depending on the extent of the placental detachment, the consequences to baby could range from nothing, to fetal distress, to brain damage, to death.

The incidence of placental abruption is about 1 in 100 births. Placental abruption is usually caused by conditions or situations that are due to reduced blood flow to the placenta. Constricted blood vessels that reduce the blood flow to the placenta build up pressure within the uterus and cause the placenta to detach. The following risk factors are known to be closely associated with reduced blood supply to the placenta:

- high blood pressure
- smoking
- cocaine or amphetamine use
- abdominal trauma
- maternal age over thirty-five
- prior pregnancy with abruption

- sickle cell anemia
- more than one pregnancy and delivery

Unfortunately, placental abruption can also occur without any of these risk factors, for unknown reasons. The diagnosis of placental abruption is usually made by observing mother's rigid and painful abdomen, vaginal bleeding, and often noting fetal distress on the fetal monitor.

Treatment begins by obtaining medical attention and monitoring of the baby to quickly determine mother and baby's status. Blood should be made available for possible transfusion in the case of emergency hemorrhage. In mild cases, hospital observation and bed rest with special monitoring may be all that is required. More often, delivery is the treatment of choice. Delivery could be either by vaginal route or emergency C-section, depending on the status of mother's cervix and the condition of the baby within the uterus. Once delivered, the placenta is closely evaluated for signs of detachment and blood clot. On occasion, the placenta may be sent to the pathology lab for further evaluation.

11

Countdown to Delivery

As the big day nears, the excitement is almost tangible. Soon you'll be meeting your baby face to face! It's true that some women feel as if they've been expecting forever and are eager to deliver, while others have loved being pregnant and wish the experience could last a bit longer.

However you're feeling about your pregnancy, chances are you still have some pressing questions that need answering before you'll feel ready for the big event. From wondering what false contractions feel like, to contemplating how often your baby should be moving now, to worrying about the effects of overshooting your due date, sometimes it seems as if every thought is focused on your child and the delivery. That's natural! Rest assured, in the next few pages, you'll find the answers to many of your questions.

1.   How often should I feel the baby move?

As mentioned earlier, most women feel their unborn babies move for the first time at between 16 and 20 weeks. The feeling is often described as a fluttering that comes and goes quickly. Over time, the movements become stronger and more predictable. By the third trimester, fetal movement should be fairly regular and consistent. Many women notice that their babies seem to move the most at the end of the day, when mothers are trying to go to sleep. Some babies seem to be more active than others for unknown reasons. You will soon become familiar with the pattern of activity that is normal for your baby.

As a general third trimester guideline, your baby should move at least ten times during a two- or three-hour period. If you notice that your baby is not moving at this rate or the rate to which you have become accustomed, try these activities prior to calling your doctor. First, drink fruit juice or another beverage that is high in natural sugars. This usually wakes up the baby with a rush of carbohydrate and sugar energy. (Some unborn babies have sleep patterns that last for a few hours at a time.) Then situate yourself in a comfortable position either on your left or right side. Count the number of times that you feel your baby move. Movements may vary from a flutter, to a kick, to a somersault. Do this activity for one to two hours. You can be reassured if you feel the baby moving again in the normal established pattern.

If you are not reassured by the above activities, then call your physician. This is especially urgent if the following conditions apply:

- fewer than ten movements after two hours of monitoring
- no movement all day
- movement of the baby much different from yesterday

You will be asked to come to your doctor's office, or to go to the hospital for fetal monitoring. Fetal monitoring consists of a small monitor being held in place over your abdomen by an elastic strap. This will record the fetal heart rate on monitor paper. The procedure usually takes about one hour. If there is any concern about the fetal heart rate, your doctor will be notified for further evaluation.

2. What are Braxton Hicks or false labor contractions?

False labor, also known as *Braxton Hicks* contractions, may occur alone or as a precursor to true labor contractions. You may or may not experience Braxton Hicks contractions.

When you are trying to distinguish between Braxton Hicks contractions and true labor, here are some guidelines to keep in mind.

Strength of contractions:

False labor or Braxton Hicks contractions are almost always fairly weak and do not tend to change over time. True contractions continue to increase steadily in their intensity.

Timing of contractions:

False contractions usually are unpredictable and irregular in timing. True contractions are regular and continue to get closer together. True contractions typically last from thirty to seventy seconds. Often five to seven minutes pass from the beginning of the first true contraction to the beginning of the next true contraction.

Change with movement:

Braxton Hicks contractions may stop or reduce in their intensity if you walk, rest, or change position. True contractions won't change in their intensity despite your position changes.

If you are unable to tell whether your contractions are true labor call your physician for further evaluation. Ultimately, the proof of true labor and contractions is noting a change in your cervix. That can be evaluated only by pelvic examination.

3. How often will I have pelvic exams?

As mentioned earlier, a pelvic exam is usually done during your first prenatal visit. During that examination, a Pap test and tests for sexually transmitted diseases are also performed. Unless you are at high risk for other problems (twins, history of premature labor, incompetent cervix) or are experiencing symptoms (cramping, bleeding, unusual discharge), no other pelvic exams are normally done until the last month. Pelvic examinations are then typically performed each week until delivery.

The first pelvic exam done in your last month of pregnancy is especially important. This is the time when many doctors perform the culture swab for Group B strep infection. As mentioned earlier, this is an important test for the future health of the newborn. Additionally, your health care provider can usually determine which part of the baby is presenting toward the opening of your cervix. Ideally, the baby's head will be in the downward position and ready for the upcoming delivery. If there is any question about the position of the baby, an ultrasound may be ordered at this time.

The other important information derived from the pelvic examination is the status of your cervix. It tells the *dilation* and *effacement* of your cervix. The cervical opening is a tiny round hole that is usually almost completely closed. For a vaginal delivery, the cervix must dilate to a size of 10 centimeters. The concept of effacement is slightly more difficult to understand. Imagine that you are not pregnant and are able to look at or feel your cervix. It actually looks and feels something like your nose. Most cervixes are firm and measure 3 or 4 centimeters in length. When you become pregnant, over time your cervix begins to soften and slightly shorten. This is due to the weight of the pregnancy, occasional contractions, and loss of mucus. By the time you near your last month of pregnancy, your cervix has changed considerably. Your cervix that was once 4 centimeters may now be perhaps only 2 centimeters in length. Since it is now approximately half the length of a normal nonpregnant cervix, doctors would call this cervix 50 percent effaced. Just as in the case of cervical dilation, the more effaced your cervix becomes, the more your cervix is ready for active labor. Determining effacement is not an exact science, and that's why different health providers often come up with different percentages. However, all agree that this process will continue gradually before or during labor until your cervix becomes completely thin and 100 percent effaced for the delivery. Therefore, by the time you are ready to push, your cervix should be 10 centimeters dilated and 100 percent effaced. Weekly pelvic exams performed in the doctor's office give you and your doctor an idea of the status of your cervix before you actually go into active labor (dilating 1 centimeter an hour). These two measurements are important to help your doctor determine your chances of going into active labor.

4. What happens if my baby is in a breech position?

By the time you reach 36 weeks of pregnancy, most fetuses will be in the head-down position. However, about 3 percent of fetuses will be in a *breech position*. That means that either the baby's buttocks or feet are in a position to be delivered first.

Most doctors do not recommend a vaginal breech delivery because of the potential dangers. This is especially true if it is your first vaginal delivery. Breech vaginal deliveries are considered high-risk because the head is the last part of the baby to be delivered. Since the head is the largest and firmest part of the baby, it could become stuck or be difficult to deliver. The resulting lack of oxygen to the baby could result in brain damage or death.

Certain risk factors make a breech presentation more likely:

- abnormally shaped uterus
- too much or too little amniotic fluid
- twins or triplets
- certain birth defects
- history of more than one pregnancy and delivery
- placenta previa
- premature labor

Despite these risk factors, sometimes a baby may be in a breech position for unknown reasons.

The position of the baby is diagnosed by examining the pregnant woman's abdomen, performing a pelvic exam, and sometimes using ultrasound to confirm the position.

If your baby is in a breech position, discuss your delivery options with your doctor. Some doctors provide handouts on exercises that you may wish to try at home in the hope of causing your unborn baby to rotate.

Another option is called a *version*. Versions have about a 50 percent success rate. The procedure is performed in the hospital; one or two doctors place their hands on your pregnant abdomen and manually attempt to push and turn the baby into the head-down position.

Naturally, pain tolerance varies among individuals, but many women report that this is a very uncomfortable procedure. Talk with your doctor about the pros and cons of this practice.

Your other option is to schedule a planned C-section for your baby's delivery. Usually the surgery is performed about one week prior to the original due date. This is done to reduce the chances of your going into labor when the baby is in the breech position.

5.   Can I deliver my baby at home?

Some women visualize delivering their babies in the comfortable surroundings of home. It is much more appealing than the sterile and unknown environment of a hospital. However, this can be risky. Many events occur during the birthing process. Most of them are natural and not harmful. However, some of these events could seriously jeopardize you or your baby. In the home setting, you are not prepared to deal with these emergent situations. Although they may not happen, should any of them occur, it could be disastrous for you or your baby.

The advantages of home delivery include:

- familiar, comfortable environment
- family and friends
- more freedom during labor
- little or no cost
- reduced chance of tearing because no instruments are used
- natural, en vogue, popular thing to do

It's true that nothing can compare to the comforts of your own home and bed. Being surrounded by as many friends and family as you desire is also a nice option for you. It's great to have the freedom to eat, move about, and do exactly as you like during labor. Certainly, the cost of a home delivery is minimal, being limited to hired personnel such as a lay midwife or doula. Certain celebrities and a handful of other influential women have stated that home birth is the natural and best way to have a baby and insist that it's been done this way successfully for centuries. Unfortunately, many, many home deliveries have also resulted in death to either mother, baby, or both.

The majority of people, especially those in the medical profession, believe that a hospital delivery is the safest form of delivery for you and your baby. Many medical professionals have come to this conclusion because they have seen firsthand the poor outcomes of failed home deliveries. Disadvantages of home birth include:

For the Baby:
- fetal distress
- infection
- too big to deliver vaginally
- breech or other abnormal presentation
- birth defect undiagnosed prior to delivery

For the Mother:
- no option of pain control
- infection
- severe bleeding

The major disadvantage of home birth is that medical personnel and technology are not available to care for the baby or the mother should an emergency arise. There are no adequate home monitors to accurately diagnose fetal distress or infection. Even if there were, the home is not equipped for any emergent action that might be required.

Also, after many hours of labor, it may become apparent that the baby is too large to deliver vaginally and is stuck in the birth canal. Sometimes it is discovered that the baby is breech or is in another type of unusual presentation such that a C-section is the baby's safest mode of delivery. Finally, once the baby is born, it may be discovered that the baby has a previously undiagnosed birth defect requiring immediate medical attention.

For the mother, the problems associated with a home birth are usually less dramatic than those for the baby. For example, she may change her mind and decide that she desires pain medication after all. While doing without that is extremely uncomfortable and agonizing, it is not life-threatening. However, infection or extremely heavy bleeding could become serious medical concerns for the mother. Infection could spread throughout her pelvis and enter her bloodstream, with serious medical consequences. Bleeding could occur if the uterus fails to stop bleeding after delivery, the placenta fails to detach, or there are unseen tears and lacerations. Any of these conditions require professional expertise for evaluation and management. Too often these situations can lead to the home birth patient and her entourage desperately coming to the hospital in the midst of a dire emergency.

Fortunately, severe and life-threatening emergencies don't happen often. However, if they do, only a hospital will provide you with the expertise to optimally handle the situation.

6. When is labor induction desirable?

Induction of labor is defined as an action or medication that puts you into labor before your body would otherwise go into labor on its own. About 15 percent of pregnant women in the United States have their labor induced by their health providers.

Your doctor may recommend labor induction under the following circumstances:

- high blood pressure, preeclampsia

- diabetes or other medical problems
- infection in uterus
- placental abruption
- water broken, but no contractions
- history of short labor and long drive to hospital

Depending on how dilated and effaced your cervix is, there are a number of ways for the doctor to induce your labor. If your cervix is dilated 2 or 3 centimeters and is at least 50 percent effaced, induction will likely be an easy process. However, if your cervix is closed and thick, several methods may be necessary over a few days to prepare your cervix for labor. Talk with your doctor about which of these common methods of inducing labor is best for you.

Mechanical Device (Foley Bulb or Laminaria)

The Foley bulb is a small balloon-like device that is inserted into your cervix while deflated and then inflated to about 1 centimeter. It is usually kept in your cervix for several hours or until it falls out. Similarly, the laminaria resembles a small thin twig made of seaweed. Several laminaria are soaked in water and placed in your cervix. Over a few hours they expand and slowly dilate your cervix to about 1 centimeter. They typically stay in a few hours or until they fall out. Both methods feel similar to a pelvic exam and are used to soften and ripen the cervix when it is not yet ready to dilate or efface easily on its own. Neither procedure poses risk to the baby, and both are almost always performed in the doctor's office.

Stripping Membranes

Part of a pelvic exam, this method is used to stretch and stimulate a cervix that is already somewhat dilated and seems ready to further dilate and efface easily on its own. This procedure is almost always done in the doctor's office. It is performed by the examiner doing a pelvic exam and sweeping his or her finger over the membranes during the pelvic exam. There is no danger to the baby.

Breaking Bag of Water (Membranes)

This procedure is always performed in the hospital for safety reasons because it requires fetal monitoring. It is performed by the doctor with a small plastic hook during a pelvic exam. The artificial rupturing of membranes is usually done when the cervix seems ripe and ready to deliver. The act of rupturing the membranes usually causes the uterus to contract. Once the bag of water is broken, the general guideline is to deliver the baby within the next twenty-four hours to reduce the chance of infection.

IV Pitocin

Pitocin is a special medication that causes the uterus to contract. It is often given in conjunction with breaking the bag of water. It is typically used when the cervix is ripe and ready for labor. This is always given in the hospital for safety reasons, because it requires fetal monitoring.

Prostaglandin by Mouth or Vagina

Prostaglandin tablets may be used either when the cervix seems ready for labor or as a prelude, when the cervix is still thick and firm. Tablets may be taken orally or suppositories may be placed within the vagina. This is always done in the hospital for safety reasons, since it also requires fetal monitoring.

Especially if your cervix is ripe and ready for labor, there is very little risk associated with labor induction. Very rarely, fetal distress or uterine rupture may occur. In the very unlikely event of emergency, an urgent C-section could be required.

7. How safe is it to go past my due date?

Your due date is calculated as 40 weeks from your last period. Very few women deliver exactly on their due dates. Most women deliver at between 37 and 42 weeks. Once you reach 42 weeks, there are increased risks to the baby:

- placenta old and calcified, reduces oxygen and nutrients to baby
- less amniotic fluid, increased chance of cord compression that reduces baby's oxygen and nutrients
- meconium passage, increasing chance of aspiration at birth (Meconium is the greenish stool in the bowels of a fetus, usually passed after delivery.)
- dysmaturity syndrome (malnourished body with long hair and nails, wrinkly skin, "little old man" appearance)
- large baby
- increased C-section rate

Because it is preferable to avoid these problems, many doctors recommend inducing labor at 41 or 42 weeks. Other reasons to induce include diabetes, preeclampsia, or other medical problems.

If you are not induced, then additional fetal assessment will be required. Fetal assessment is important to ensure that the fetus is healthy and doing well inside the uterus. The two tests most commonly performed are the twice-weekly non-stress test (monitoring fetal heart rate and movement) and the weekly ultrasound to measure the volume of amniotic fluid. If these two tests are reassuring, it greatly increases confidence about the well-being of the fetus. Another test that is sometimes performed is called a *biophysical profile*. This is a special type of ultrasound that examines the baby's organ systems to determine fetal well-being.

12

Cesarean Sections (C-sections)

You may very well be planning a natural childbirth. Or you may be among those patients who know ahead of time that they have a specific medical condition, requiring a C-section. Women carrying twins or triplets, those with a breech baby, and those with maternal diabetes are much more likely to have C-sections. However, some women do not know that they will deliver by C-section until they have experienced at least several hours of labor. This chapter explains when and why C-sections are required.

1. Why might I need a C-section?

A *Cesarean section,* or *C-section,* is a surgical method of delivering the baby through an incision in your lower abdomen. Certain medical conditions make a C-section the safest choice for delivering your baby.

In some cases, these conditions are known in advance and the surgery can be prearranged. In other cases, the situation may not become entirely apparent until the mother has experienced some portion of labor.

When a woman knows that she has a condition requiring a C-section, she can plan for it in advance. Scheduled C-sections are typically performed approximately one week prior to the due date.

Cesarean Sections (C-sections)

They are performed early in an attempt to prevent the mother from going into labor. Reasons for scheduled C-sections include:

- breech; failed or declined version
- placenta previa
- previous C-section; declined trial of labor
- herpes outbreak within seven to ten days of projected delivery date
- multiple fetuses (C-section for twins depends on the position of the babies in the uterus at the time of delivery. All other multiple fetuses are delivered by scheduled C-section.)
- maternal diabetes (Diabetes is associated with extremely large babies. If the baby is approximately 9-1/2 to 10 pounds or more on ultrasound, plans for a C-section are made.)

In unplanned cases of C-section, the mother first experiences labor. After a varying number of hours, it may eventually become clear that a vaginal delivery is no longer the best and safest form of delivery for the baby. Reasons for unplanned C-sections include:

- fetal distress; non-reassuring heartbeat
- umbilical cord compression; reduced blood flow to baby
- baby not able to fit through mother's pelvis
- labor and contractions stop, cervix fails to dilate further
- twins; failed vaginal delivery

The incision made to deliver the baby by C-section is usually low, horizontal ("bikini"), and often through or just above the (shaved) pubic hair region. The entire C-section procedure takes only about one hour to perform. Postoperative recovery is usually three days in the hospital and two to three weeks at home.

A vaginal delivery is almost everyone's preference. However, a vaginal delivery may not always be the best and safest route of delivery for your baby. The C-section offers a safe birthing alternative in certain situations. The most important goal is always the health and safety of mother and baby.

2. If I've had a previous C-section, how should my new baby be delivered?

When deciding whether you will deliver vaginally or by C-section if you've had a previous C-section, you and your doctor will want to consider several factors. Among them are the type of incision made on your uterus during your previous C-section, the position of the baby's head, the condition of the cervix as the delivery nears, reasons for your first C-section, and your future childbearing plans.

The type of incision made in your uterus during your first C-section is a major factor when considering how to have your next child. (By the way, the incision made in your skin is not necessarily the same type of incision made in your uterus.) If you are unsure of the type of incision made, your doctor may want to review your previous surgical records. Horizontal incisions are the more common type of incision made. However, occasionally a vertical incision becomes necessary. If a vertical incision was made during your first C-section, your incision may not be strong enough to endure contractions and your doctor will probably recommend a repeat C-section. The purpose of a repeat C-section is to avoid the chance of uterine rupture. Uterine rupture can cause serious medical problems for mother and baby, including bleeding, fetal distress, and death. (There is a small chance that uterine rupture could occur with a prior horizontal incision, but the chances are about ten times greater with vertical uterine incisions.)

Assuming that your past uterine incision was horizontal, it is largely up to you to decide whether you wish to schedule a repeat C-section or want to attempt to deliver vaginally. A vaginal delivery after C-section is called a *VBAC*, which stands for *vaginal birth after cesarean*. Your chances of a successful VBAC are greatest if your baby's head is deep into your pelvis and your cervix is ripe with good dilation and effacement as your due date nears. A repeat C-section avoids the chance of uterine rupture, while a VBAC holds a slight risk.

The reason you had your first C-section is also important to consider when deciding your method of delivery this time. How likely is this condition to occur again? For example, if your first C-section was necessary because your pelvis was too small, this may very well be the case again. However, if it was because of fetal distress, a herpes outbreak, breech, twins, or abnormal placenta, the condition may be less likely to reoccur during the second labor.

Another consideration should be your plans for future child-bearing. If you plan to have several more children, a vaginal delivery may be preferable so you can avoid multiple C-sections. Conversely, if you know that this is your last baby, you may elect to have a tubal ligation procedure at the time of your scheduled repeat C-section and avoid any additional procedures later.

You and your doctor will discuss the pros and cons of repeat C-section versus VBAC. Infection and bleeding are rare, but are more likely to occur with any surgical procedure, including repeat C-section. Anesthesia risks can be encountered with either form of delivery and are always low. A repeat C-section usually involves an epidural-like anesthetic. Similarly, many VBAC patients in labor desire a laboring epidural. You and your family and friends will be more involved in the delivery if it is a vaginal delivery. C-sections are performed in the sterile environment of the operating room. Family and friends are usually limited to one or two in the room with you.

Try not to let the pain of labor play a role in your decision. Pain can be controlled by other measures other than having an epidural with a C-section. Besides, whatever pain you might miss by avoiding labor, you will probably make up with postoperative pain and discomfort. Your recovery will be somewhat longer and more painful with a C-section. Most women report moderate discomfort for a few days, subsiding substantially after that. Also remember that you may opt for a

VBAC and it could still be unsuccessful. In that case, you could end up having a repeat C-section after all.

3. Must I have a C-section if I'm carrying twins?

Not necessarily. It's true that your risk of having a C-section is higher with twins than with a single baby; however, there is an excellent chance that a C-section may not be necessary. The decision to deliver vaginally or by C-section is determined largely by the position of the twins within your uterus. As delivery time nears, the majority of twins are both in the head-down position. This is an ideal position for a vaginal delivery. Some doctors may also agree to a vaginal delivery if the first twin is head-down, regardless of the position of the second twin. Others will recommend a C-section if the babies' positions are anything other than both heads-down. Certainly if the first twin is breech or transverse (sideways), a C-section is almost always recommended.

Vaginal twin delivery is often done in a double setup environment. That means the delivery takes place in an operating room and preparations for both a vaginal delivery and a C-section are made. The patient sits in the birthing bed and preparations are made for a vaginal delivery. However, on the other side of the room, a complete operating room staff and equipment are standing by in case an urgent C-section is needed. A C-section could be performed to deliver both babies, or only to deliver the second baby. The double setup is strictly a precautionary measure.

Another important consideration when considering the mode of delivery is whether you or the twins have additional medical issues. Twin pregnancies have a higher incidence of prematurity, growth abnormalities, birth defects, maternal diabetes, preeclampsia, and placental abnormalities. Any of these factors could increase your risk for having a C-section.

4. If I have a C-section, will you tie my tubes if I wish?

Almost all doctors will perform a *tubal ligation* (cutting and tying the fallopian tubes for permanent sterilization) simultaneously with your C-section if you wish. However, be sure to speak to your doctor about this issue early during your prenatal visits. Discuss the permanence and finality of the decision with your doctor and your partner. It may be true that in rare cases, permanent sterilization can be reversed. However, this is costly (insurance won't pay) and painful (requires another operation), and is not guaranteed to be successful. Do not elect to have permanent sterilization unless you are absolutely certain that you are finished with childbearing.

Once you've thought it through and decided to have your tubes tied, let your doctor know so he or she can document that choice on your medical record. If you decide at the last minute or during labor that you desire permanent sterilization, many doctors will not perform the procedure. That's because they are concerned that either the narcotic pain medication or the labor pain itself has affected your decision. Some studies have shown an increase in guilt, regret, and postpartum depression in women who have sterilization procedures that were not well thought out.

Some doctors will not perform permanent sterilization procedures because of their religious beliefs. Hospitals with certain religious affiliations may not permit the procedure to be done. Ideally, you have already had a complete discussion about these issues at the beginning of your pregnancy, when you were selecting your physician and hospital. If that was not done or you want to reconfirm, be sure to have a conversation with your physician about these issues before you go into labor.

Part IV
Labor and Delivery

13

Going to the Hospital

It's almost the big day! Over the years, you've no doubt seen movies in which pregnant women exclaim to their mates, "It's time!" They grab the waiting suitcase and race to the hospital. Soon, you'll be the one grabbing the suitcase and heading for the hospital for the birth of your baby. But you may not need to race to the hospital as quickly as you might think. This chapter will help you understand the signs of labor and when it's time to go to the hospital. In the meantime, during your remaining prenatal visits, be sure to clarify with your doctor how he or she wants you to handle these situations:

- When should you call the doctor?
- What do you do if the office is closed?
- Should you call the doctor before going to the hospital?

Realize that only about 5 percent of women actually deliver on their due dates. Most women deliver at between 37 and 42 weeks. There is no truth to the old saying that a first baby is always past due. So be prepared a little bit early, just in case!

1. How do I know when to go to the hospital?

You will probably be more comfortable in your own home during the early stages of labor. Unless you have a known high-risk condition or have been told otherwise, most doctors encourage their patients to stay home during early labor. Eventually you will need to go to the hospital for medical evaluation depending on the status of your contractions, amniotic fluid, and (if applicable) bleeding.

Labor Contractions

True labor contractions occur approximately every five minutes and last for one minute. The contractions should be so painful that you cannot walk or talk through them. True contractions cause your abdomen to become as firm as your forehead. Changing your activity (resting, showering, walking) does not stop them. Once these regular and strong contractions have gone on for one to two hours, you should go to the hospital. If you are unsure whether the contractions are real versus early or false labor, you should still go to the hospital for evaluation.

Leaking Amniotic Fluid

If your amniotic fluid (bag of water) breaks, you should prepare to go to the hospital. If your fluid is clear and your Group B strep status is negative, you can usually wait six to eight hours before going to the hospital. Ask your doctor for his or her policy on this matter. Most of the time, labor contractions will begin within a few hours and you will want to go to the hospital anyway. On the other hand, if your amniotic fluid is a brownish-green color or your Group B strep status is positive, then you should go to the hospital immediately.

Bleeding

It is quite common to have a scant amount of spotting after sex, exercise, or a pelvic exam. However, if you are bleeding more than a few teaspoons of bright red blood, you should go to the hospital for further evaluation and treatment. You should also go to the hospital if the bleeding is accompanied by severe abdominal pain.

Some doctors prefer that you call their office or answering service first, before heading to the hospital. That way, the doctor can discuss your symptoms with you. If you and the doctor agree that it's time for you go to the hospital, the doctor usually calls the hospital to notify them and make preparations for your arrival. Other doctors prefer that you to go to the hospital for evaluation first, and then have the hospital staff call the doctor with a report on your condition. Both methods are perfectly acceptable. Be sure to ask your doctor his or her office policy.

Here's one last word of advice about getting to the hospital: In an emergency, never drive yourself to the hospital. Always have a spouse, partner, family member, or friend take you.

If you are alone in an emergency, the safest way to get to the hospital is to call 911 and wait for paramedic assistance. This may seem like an extreme measure; however, it's always best to err on the side of caution when the health of mother and baby are involved.

2.   What is a mucus plug and what does it indicate?

From the time of early pregnancy, a protective mucus coating builds up over your cervix. This mucus provides additional protection to the growing fetus inside your uterus. As your due date nears, your cervix begins to gradually prepare for delivery with mild dilation and effacement. As the cervix goes through these changes, part of the mucus becomes loosened and is discharged through your vagina. It may be clear and sticky; it may look jelly-like; sometimes it is blood-tinged. Mucus discharge (sometimes called bloody show), often with some degree of blood tinge, is a gradual process that occurs over several days or weeks. Many people are under the impression that the mucus is in the shape of a plug, much like a cork. They think that once a bit of mucus is out, no additional mucus will be discharged. In reality, that is usually not the case.

If you are 36 weeks along or more in your pregnancy, mucus discharge or bloody show is completely normal. There is no reason to call your doctor. It is merely a sign that your cervix is preparing for the upcoming delivery. However, if your due date is more than one month away and you are experiencing excessive mucus or bloody show, call your doctor, because this could be a sign of preterm labor.

3. What should I take to the hospital?

The hospital labor and delivery unit has everything you need to deliver your baby. Most modern hospitals go to great lengths to provide an optimum birthing experience. However, you will still want to bring certain items with you to make your environment more comfortable and your birthing experience more personal. Here is a list of items to consider when packing for the hospital:

- familiar objects to soothe you; music, pillows, pictures
- robe and socks or slippers
- camera or video camera (check batteries)
- calling card, phone numbers to call family and friends
- toiletries
- nursing nightgown (if breast-feeding)
- nursing bra and breast pads (if breast-feeding)
- baby hat and booties
- receiving blankets
- infant car seat
- baby's homecoming outfit

It's a good idea to have these items assembled and ready to go approximately two to three weeks prior to your due date, in case labor occurs early.

14

At the Hospital

The days of not being able to see your feet are almost over! Whether you're coming to the hospital because your water broke, you're in labor, or it just feels like it's the right time, arriving at the hospital is a big event. After all the months of planning and dreaming, motherhood is now just a birthing room away.

So much is about to happen, so quickly. Soon, you'll be holding your new baby in your arms! These next few hours will be among the most memorable in your entire life.

1. What is a birthing room?

The *birthing room* is the room in the hospital where you will labor and eventually deliver your baby. After the delivery, you and your baby will recover in this room. In some hospitals you stay in this same room until you are discharged to your home a couple of days later. In other hospitals, you are moved from the birthing room to a different room about one to two hours after your delivery. In this case, you will spend the remaining couple of days in your postpartum recovery room.

When you initially come to the hospital for medical evaluation, you are usually taken to a holding area for monitoring and evaluation. This holding area is called the *triage unit.* While in the triage unit, you and the baby are assessed for signs of labor and fetal well-being. If you are in labor or any problems are detected, you will be admitted and sent to your birthing room for further observation.

Modern hospitals go out of their way to make the birthing room environment as homey and comfortable as possible. They know that they cannot replicate your own home, but most try very hard to give you many amenities and comforts for an optimal birthing experience within the confines and safety of a hospital setting. Some of the amenities found in modern birthing rooms include microwave ovens, coffeemakers, recliners, tasteful decor, cable television, Jacuzzi bathtubs, gentle lighting, and a family-centered environment. Within the same room and hidden discreetly in ceilings and behind walls is the medical equipment necessary to handle almost any emergency. Central fetal monitoring is located at the nurse's station just outside of your door, so that a medical professional is always watching your baby's heart rate and your contractions. If necessary, additional portable equipment can be brought into your room or you can be transported to the operating room should a C-section become necessary.

2. Will I be shaved? Will I receive an enema in the hospital?

For a vaginal delivery, hospital shaving and enemas are things of the past. Your pubic region will be partially shaved if you are having a C-section. Even then, the shaving is minimal and involves only the area of the surgical incision.

Enemas are available and you may have one if you desire, but they are no longer performed routinely for either vaginal or C-section delivery. You may want to know that many women have bowel movements during labor and almost always when they are pushing.

This is completely normal because of the pelvic muscles involved. If you think that this will bother or embarrass you, then speak with your doctor about having an enema while you are still in the early stages of labor.

3. How many monitors and tubes must I be attached to during labor?

When you first arrive at the hospital, the nurse will take your blood pressure and pulse, and then attach two straps to your abdomen to monitor the baby's heart rate and your contractions. Usually the hospital has a policy that you must undergo this monitoring for a certain amount of time (for example, twenty minutes to one hour) to ensure that the baby is safely handling the stress of your contractions. Your blood pressure and medical history will also be reviewed to see if additional care, tests, or monitors are needed. For example, if you have preeclampsia, you will be confined to bed; if you have gestational diabetes, then blood sugars will be checked during labor.

Once the medical staff has assessed that your situation is safe, many mothers opt to remove the monitors and enjoy some mobility. You may walk around your room or hospital floor, take a shower or bath, or sit in a comfortable chair. Other mothers may want to receive pain medication immediately, or need intravenous (IV) antibiotics due to a positive Group B strep. These women will have limited mobility and require additional monitoring.

Fetal Monitoring

This type of monitoring is always required for at least a portion of your labor. The purpose of fetal monitoring is to ensure that the baby is healthy and tolerating the stresses of your uterine contractions. Monitoring may be either intermittent or continuous. Most hospitals have policies on monitoring the fetal heartbeat depending on various conditions. For example, you may need continuous fetal monitoring if you are high-risk, have a medical problem, or are being induced. If you are low-risk and have no problems, intermittent fetal monitoring may be an option. Continuous fetal monitoring requires that you stay in bed or a nearby chair. Intermittent monitoring is more flexible and allows you some degree of mobility. Fetal monitoring may be done externally or internally. A wide elastic belt is placed around your abdomen to hold the external fetal monitor in place. With internal monitoring, a small electrode is attached to the baby's scalp.

Uterine Contraction Monitoring

It is important for the medical staff to monitor the relationship between your baby's heart rate and your contractions. Certain patterns develop between the baby's heart rate and your uterine contractions. Some patterns are reassuring and represent fetal well-being. On the other hand, certain patterns between the baby's heart rate and uterine contractions can indicate fetal distress. As with fetal monitoring, contractions may be monitored either externally or internally. A wide elastic belt is placed around your abdomen to hold the external uterine contraction monitor in place. With internal monitoring, your bag of water must be broken and a small straw-like catheter device is placed inside the uterus; it lies freely between the baby and the wall of your uterus. Internal monitoring is used in high-risk situations or with problems that require more cautious observation.

Intravenous (IV) Lines

Intravenous (IV) lines are not always required. However, most women seem to end up with one. You need an IV line if you want pain medication or an epidural, need antibiotics, need other specialized medications, or if there are signs of fetal distress. If you are having a C-section, you definitely will need an IV.

Foley Catheter

A catheter, a tube in the bladder to drain urine, is not used routinely for a vaginal delivery. However, you will need a Foley catheter in your bladder if you have a C-section or if you decide to have an epidural during labor. In either case, you won't be able to feel the catheter in your bladder because you'll be numb in that area.

It's important to have an empty bladder during a C-section because the bladder and the uterus are very close to one another. The Foley catheter keeps the bladder completely drained and out of the way of the surgical field. It is much easier and safer to make an incision in the uterus when the bladder is empty.

It's convenient to have a Foley catheter when you have a labor epidural. Because the bottom half of your body is numb, you aren't able to get up and walk to the bathroom. You probably also can't tell when you have a full bladder. If your bladder becomes very full, the baby's head may have a difficult time descending into your pelvis. The Foley catheter solves this problem by keeping the bladder drained and providing additional room for the baby's head to descend into the pelvis.

Oxygen Mask

An oxygen mask is rarely needed. It may be a treatment option if the fetus needs extra oxygen, as in the case of fetal distress.

4. Can I eat during labor?

Many women find that they are not very hungry during labor. Usually the combination of contraction pain and occasional nausea is enough to reduce your appetite. However, do ask your doctor about his or her policy on eating during labor. Many doctors will okay your having light foods or clear liquids (Popsicles, Jell-O, or broth). Other doctors recommend only water and ice chips.

There are two main concerns with eating during labor. The first is that you may become nauseated and vomit during the labor or delivery process. Naturally, this is uncomfortable for you and distracts from your birthing experience.

The other reason to limit your intake relates to the possibility of an emergency C-section. You probably know that most surgeries are performed when the patient has an empty stomach (nothing to eat or drink for eight to twelve hours prior). When you are pregnant, your digestive system is slowed and it takes even longer to empty your stomach. If you are eating during labor and for some reason need an urgent C-section, your stomach will not be empty. Having food in your stomach increases your chance of aspiration during surgery. Aspiration occurs when food particles are regurgitated upward and go down your windpipe (trachea) and into your lungs. This can result in very serious infectious pneumonia, severe breathing difficulties, or even death. Fortunately, all of these are very unlikely occurrences. However, in the event that a C-section is necessary, anesthesia is safer if your stomach is empty.

5. How many family and friends can be in the room for the delivery?

Ask both your doctor and your hospital about policies regarding your visiting family members and friends. Most doctors and hospitals are quite lenient because they want to foster comfortable and homey surroundings for the birthing family. In most cases, you may have as many adult family members and friends in the room as you like. Children, however, may or may not be allowed. Be advised that children under the age of twelve may be banned from certain areas of the hospital, including maternity, the nursery, and intensive care, during the flu and cold season. That's because during these winter months, a virus called respiratory syncytial virus (RSV) is often spread among school-age children. This very potent virus can cause a serious form of pneumonia in newborns.

If you are having a C-section, there is a greater chance that you will be limited in the number of family members and friends who can accompany you into the operating room. Operating room guests are generally limited to one or two family members or friends.

In the rare case of an emergency, visitors will probably be asked to leave the room so that medical personnel can perform their necessary tasks most efficiently.

6. What are the stages of labor and how long do they take?

There are three stages of labor: labor contractions, pushing, and the delivery of the placenta (the afterbirth).

Stage 1

The first stage begins with the onset of contractions and cervical dilation, and ends when your cervix is fully dilated. This is generally considered the most painful and the longest of the three stages. If this is your first baby, average time for the first stage is about ten hours. For a second baby the average time is reduced to about six hours. Generally, cervix dilation between 1 and 3 centimeters is considered early labor. Many women spend this time at home, walking around, showering, and preparing to go to the hospital. *Cervical dilation* between 4 and 6 centimeters is the active phase. By this time, most women are settled into the hospital and many request pain relief. Cervical dilation between 7 and 9 centimeters is commonly called transition. It is accompanied by even more intense contractions, bouts of vomiting, and a feeling of pressure as the baby's head descends deeper into your pelvis. Finally, at 10 centimeters, your cervix is completely dilated and you are ready to begin pushing. Most women feel a strong desire to push and describe the sensation as if they desperately need to have a bowel movement. Every labor is different. A good rule of thumb for a first baby is that you will dilate about 1 centimeter per hour. You can't start pushing until you reach 10 centimeters. So if you start out at 2 centimeters, once you are in active labor, you will likely be ready to push in about eight hours.

Naturally, there are exceptions to this; some women proceed with lightning speed and others have long, drawn-out labors.

Stage II

Stage two is the pushing phase. It begins once your cervix is fully dilated and ends with the delivery of the baby. Many women feel a sense of relief when they get to this phase. Many say that it feels good to push. If you have an epidural, you will probably need a little extra coaching to coordinate your pushing muscles. For a first baby, this phase usually lasts about one to two hours; for a second baby it is reduced to about thirty minutes.

Stage III

Stage three is the delivery of the placenta (afterbirth). It begins with the delivery of the baby and ends when the placenta has been delivered. As discussed earlier, the placenta is the life support system for the baby while it is in your uterus. When the baby has been delivered and the cord has been cut, the remainder of the cord and the attached placenta are still inside your body. Usually within ten to fifteen minutes after the baby's birth, the placenta expels itself through your vagina. The placenta is relatively large (about the size of a regular round cake) but very soft and malleable. It is attached to the baby's sac and umbilical cord. There is no pain associated with a normal placenta delivery. This feeling of passing the placenta surprises many women and some are fearful that something has gone wrong. On the other hand, many women are so preoccupied with their new babies, that they don't even notice this phase of the birthing process.

7. How often are pelvic exams done when I'm in labor?

A pelvic exam is typically done when you initially arrive at the hospital. The pelvic exam establishes the dilation and effacement of your cervix. It is also a check to determine whether your membrane (bag of water) has ruptured. The labor nurse or medical resident may assist your doctor by performing the pelvic exam and calling him or her with your progress. The pelvic exam is usually done in the hospital's labor and delivery triage area. If you are in labor, you will be sent to your own birthing room. If you are not in labor, you will be sent home.

If it cannot be easily determined whether you are in labor, you may be observed in the triage area for a couple of hours and reexamined periodically until your labor status becomes clear.

Once you are in labor, you may not have another pelvic exam until you request pain relief, want to push, or have passed several hours with seemingly few contractions. As long as labor seems to be progressing naturally and without problems, pelvic exams are usually limited. If there is a problem or concern, additional pelvic exams may be needed to assess and treat the situation.

8. What is meconium and is it dangerous?

Meconium is the baby's first stool. It is a greenish substance that is in the baby's intestines and is usually passed shortly after the baby is born. Sometimes, the baby passes meconium while it is still inside the uterus. Meconium passage prior to birth may be caused by stress, being overdue, or other medical problems. Meconium stains the amniotic fluid a greenish color. Depending on the quantity of the meconium, the amniotic fluid may range from a light green, watery liquid to a thick, pea-soup appearance. The thicker the fluid, the more potentially dangerous it is for the baby.

If the meconium staining is noted to be very light green and watery, no special treatment may be required. However, if moderate or thick meconium is noted, a special suction device and a high-risk nurse practitioner will be present at the delivery. Once the baby's head has been delivered, the airways (nose, mouth, and throat) will be suctioned with a special suction device to remove any meconium that is present. Under these circumstances, your partner is not usually allowed to cut the baby's umbilical cord and the baby is not usually placed upon your abdomen. Instead, the baby is immediately handed to the nurse resuscitator, who will thoroughly assess the baby and check the baby's airways. The goal is to avoid meconium aspiration. If the baby has aspirated meconium, this could lead to pneumonia and breathing difficulties requiring days or weeks in the intensive care nursery. This evaluation is performed in the birthing room and once the baby has been cleared, usually in only about five minutes, the baby is then handed to the parents without any further delay.

Some studies have shown that diluting the moderate and thick meconium-stained fluid with sterile saline solution may be helpful. In this situation, an internal catheter is placed inside the uterus (the same type used to monitor uterine contractions internally). The catheter is used to introduce sterile saline fluid that flushes out or dilutes the meconium-stained fluid. Some reports indicate that this procedure may minimize the risk of meconium aspiration.

9. Should my water break naturally, or should the doctor do it?

A pregnant woman has about a 30 percent chance of her water breaking by itself without the presence of contractions or someone breaking it for her. Most women's water breaks during hard labor or when the doctor ruptures the membranes during a pelvic exam. In any case, since there are no nerve endings in the bag of water, it is not a painful experience.

When a woman's water breaks it may consist of several cups of fluid or just a small trickle. Some women compare it to a water balloon bursting, while others say it feels like they are urinating on themselves. No one knows exactly what causes the membranes to rupture. It may occur while sitting, standing, or sleeping. If you are not already in labor when your water breaks, you will probably begin to experience contractions within six hours. For that reason, ruptured membranes are known to initiate and expedite the delivery process.

If a woman's labor is progressing normally and naturally, most doctors do not intervene, allowing the bag of water to break naturally. However, if there is a medical concern, the doctor may elect to artificially break the water to better scrutinize the fetal heartbeat and uterine contractions and to note the color of the fluid. The doctor may also choose to artificially rupture your membranes as a means to induce labor. Artificial rupture of membranes is done during a pelvic exam using a long plastic device. The procedure is quick and not painful.

Artificial Rupture of Membranes

Advantages	Disadvantages
Allows observation of amniotic fluid color, check for meconium (green staining), preparation to treat	Development of infection due to prolonged rupture of membranes (18 to 24 hours)
Provides access for internal monitoring, if it becomes necessary	Rare possibility of prolapse of cord leading to fetal distress (cord comes out before the baby)
Has high success rate for inducing or augmenting labor	Very rare possibility of rupture of blood vessel in membrane causing hemorrhage and need for urgent C-section

Whether the membranes rupture spontaneously or artificially, most medical professionals agree that it is preferable to know the color of the amniotic fluid prior to the pushing phase of labor. As mentioned, if the baby has passed meconium, then special instruments and nursery staff may be needed to suction the baby's airways and closely watch the baby's breathing patterns.

The main disadvantage of ruptured membranes is that if they are ruptured for a prolonged period of time (usually 18 to 24 hours) without delivery of the infant, there is a greatly increased chance of an infection in the uterus and potential harm to the baby. In such cases, Pitocin may be used to speed up the labor process, and intravenous antibiotics are usually given to help reduce the chance of developing an infection.

10. Can my delivery be videotaped?

Almost always the answer is yes. Be sure to confirm that video-taping is acceptable to your doctor and your hospital. Many doctors request that the video equipment be set-up at the head of your bed.

Many women believe that filming from this angle provides more tasteful home movies. It also keeps the equipment away from the area where the doctor needs to be to perform the delivery. On the other hand, if you are certain that you would like your videotape filmed from the "below the waist" viewpoint, that's usually permissible, too. Just ask the doctor where your family member or friend can stand to optimize your personal goals as well as those of your doctor.

Some women designate a special friend or family member to be in charge of the videotaping. If you don't want to do that, consider bringing a tripod stand with you. That way, the video camera can be set up on the stand, leaving your spouse or partner to focus entirely on you and your delivery. Many people also bring along a regular camera for taking still shots. Remember to pack extra batteries or charge existing ones when you are packing your bag for the hospital.

15

Pain Management

If you're like many mothers-to-be, you have given plenty of thought to whether giving birth is painful. You've talked to friends, many of whom described the process as painful and others who described it as surprisingly lacking in pain.

Certainly, you've heard them say, "It was worth it." But where does that leave you? You're still wondering about pain management.

Significant controversy surrounds the subject of pain management during labor. Some women believe that they must endure the entire birthing process without any medication whatsoever, thereby having a completely "natural" experience. Other women want an epidural almost immediately to avoid any discomfort at all. The truth is that you probably won't really know what you want until you are actually in the situation. The birthing process can be full of unexpected turns of events and it's best to remain flexible in your decision making. The most important advice is to educate yourself about all of your options and to keep an open mind.

1. How will my pain be managed during labor?

Many women have expectations that their labor will happen a certain way. They have predetermined beliefs about their need for pain relief. In reality, the labor process frequently does not occur according to plan. This is especially true with a first baby.

The need or desire for pain relief during labor varies greatly from woman to woman and from labor to labor. Some labors are quick and tolerable. Others seem to drag on for many hours. Different women have different tolerances for pain. Women with supportive and nurturing coaches may need less pain relief than those without them. You probably won't know what you want until you are in labor.

The choice for pain relief in labor is entirely up to you. Only you know what you are going through and how you feel. Family and friends are there to provide encouragement and support. The medical staff is there to make sure you know your options and to provide whatever relief you desire. Pain relief during labor can be classified into four categories.

If you are considering an *epidural,* you should find out your hospital's policy on anesthesia. Many hospitals offer in-house anesthesia twenty-four hours per day. That means that if you need an epidural or require an emergent C-section, anesthesiologists are in the hospital and readily available. Other hospitals do not require their anesthesiologists to stay in the hospital. However, there is always an anesthesiologist on call and available, to be called to the hospital. Normal response time is usually less than thirty minutes.

Ask your doctor or prenatal class educator about your hospital's policy. Busy hospitals and teaching hospitals tend to have more twenty-four-hour coverage than smaller, quieter hospitals. Whether anesthesiologists are in the hospital 24/7 may not have an impact on your health or the baby's health. However, if you are in pain and request an epidural, the twenty or thirty minutes you might have to wait may seem like hours.

Remember, the two most important things you can do are to know your options and to remain open-minded. Once you are in labor, you can select the best option for you.

Methods of Pain Relief

Type of Relief	Description	Advantages	Disadvantages
Supportive or interactive (requires coach or doula)	Breathing, relaxation, focal points, massage, birthing ball, shower or Jacuzzi	Natural and drug-free No risk to mother/baby Mother alert, involved	Minimal pain relief Requires active and supportive team
Local	Numb area between vagina and rectum	No risk to mother or baby	Mother alert, involved No labor pain relief, only end of delivery relief
Narcotic	IV meds to reduce overall pain	Takes edge off pain without epidural Useful for little relief	Still have some pain Drowsy mother and baby
Epidural	Injection in back causing temporary loss of feeling from the waist down	Pain-free Able to enjoy and focus on delivery Designed to last until baby is delivered	May cause fetal heartbeat to drop Slow labor, difficult to push

2. What about hiring a doula for assistance?

The word "doula" comes from a Greek word that means "woman helping woman." Today, doulas are trained laypersons who specialize in providing informational, emotional, and physical support during labor. Some belong to a national organization called DONA (Doulas of North America). That organization requires that doulas attain a certain level of knowledge about the birthing process and abide by a certain code of conduct. Although a doula is not a trained nurse, she advises and helps the patient through the labor and delivery process. Doulas supply reassurance and comfort measures such as breathing and relaxation techniques, focus, massage, and positioning with birthing balls.

Some doulas also provide services after the baby is born, helping with postpartum issues such as breast-feeding and depression. Because doulas are not medical professionals, they do not provide prenatal care, perform pelvic exams, deliver babies, or prescribe medication.

Some studies have shown that the presence of a doula during labor significantly reduces the use of pain medication and epidural requests. Some women have reported that their doulas provided incredible amounts of support and comfort that they would not have received otherwise. Remember to keep an open mind. Even if you have a doula, it is still possible that you may desire additional pain relief or require a C-section.

Spouses and partners seem to have mixed feelings about doulas. Some like doulas because having one enables them to focus on the mother as a person, not a patient. Others don't like the "invasion" of an outside person taking over their roles as "coach." Naturally, this is something to discuss with your spouse or partner.

Years ago, a labor nurse had only one laboring patient. She or he was able to focus completely on that patient during the entire labor and delivery process, and to perform many of the tasks that doulas perform today. However, now a labor nurse may be caring for two or three patients at the same time. Thus, you may not get the one-on-one care from the nursing staff that was once available. A doula may provide that special bond. Remember, though, that she is a coach and a support person; she cannot perform the medical functions of a nurse.

Doulas charge approximately $500 to $1,000 for their services; this fee is not covered by insurance.

16

The Delivery

T he countdown is complete! This is the real thing—the birth of your baby!

If the past months have felt like Pregnancy 101, today must seem like your final! But no one can completely prepare you for what delivery will be like—not your mother, your sister, or your best friend. Each birth is unique. Still, the more you know about the possibilities that lie ahead during delivery and the measures the doctor may need to take, the more confidently you can deal with them should they arise.

When the delivery is near, the nurses, doctor and hospital staff shift into high gear, ready to help you bring your baby into the world. From telling you when to push, to dealing with complications, to signaling your partner when the cord needs to be cut, they are there to ensure the health of you and your baby.

1. What happens when it's time for my delivery?

Once you have reached full cervical dilation, it's time to begin pushing. You and your labor nurse will work together to find a comfortable and effective method that works best for you. Some women like to push while resting on their sides. Others prefer the leverage of placing their legs in stirrups and holding onto special handrails. Still others prefer to grab their own knees and pull their legs toward themselves while bearing down. Your nurse is at your bedside to assist you during your pushing. This is also the time when your doctor will come to the hospital, if he or she is not already present. Just as before, the baby's heart rate and your contractions will continue to be monitored until the baby has been delivered.

As the baby's head continues to descend, many women request that a mirror be placed so they can view baby's head to motivate their pushing. As the head continues to descend it eventually begins to crown. Crowning occurs when a portion of the baby's head is visibly bulging outward from your vagina. At this time the foot of the bed is removed and your bottom is washed with an antiseptic soapy solution. Sterile drapes are spread on your legs and under your buttocks. Your doctor puts on a fluid-protective gown and gloves. He or she stands or sits in between your legs. A small table is wheeled into the room and placed next to the doctor. It contains all the necessary instruments for the delivery. In addition to your doctor and labor nurse, at least one other nursery staff member will be in the room to care for the baby. As the baby's head continues to move toward delivery, your doctor will talk to you and provide guidance so you know when and how much to push. That way you and your doctor can work together to have a gentle and well-controlled delivery. The doctor will be using a lubricant and certain manual techniques to avoid or minimize tears. If necessary, the doctor will cut an *episiotomy*, an incision made in your perineum (the area between the vagina and the rectum) for the purpose of enlarging the outlet for delivery. Once the baby's head has been delivered, the doctor will ask you to stop pushing for just a few seconds. The doctor will take this time to suction out mucus and fluid from the baby's nose and mouth. Then the doctor will ask you for one last push, and your baby will be delivered! The baby is placed upon your abdomen so you can greet and hold your baby for the first time.

2. When and why would the doctor cut an episiotomy?

The purpose of the episiotomy is to provide additional room for the baby's head and to avoid major tearing. Years ago, routine episiotomies were cut with almost every delivery. Today, most doctors cut them only if it appears that significant additional room is required for delivery. The incision is usually made as the baby's head is crowning, bulging from your vagina and almost ready for delivery.

Sometimes it is difficult to know if an episiotomy will be needed. It depends on the size and position of the baby's head and the stretching ability of the tissue around the vagina. Many doctors and midwives use mineral oil or other lubricants to soften and moisten the area. This may assist in preventing some tears.

Delivering with an intact perineum and vagina is ideal. That rarely happens with a first baby. A small tear or abrasion is almost always preferable to an episiotomy. Small tears require only a few sutures or none at all. However, if it appears that a large jagged tear may occur, then an episiotomy, a straight surgical incision, would be preferable. An episiotomy controls the placement of the cut (midline is best) and the size and direction of the cut (avoiding the rectum is best). If it appears that an episiotomy is needed, a local anesthetic medication is injected into the area so you won't feel pain. If you have already had an epidural, the local anesthetic may not be necessary.

3. What is fetal distress and how could it affect my delivery?

During the labor and delivery process, a continuous record of the fetus's heartbeat is monitored. Normal fetal heart rate is between 110 and 160 beats per minute. If the fetal heartbeat is considerably higher or lower than the normal range, this requires evaluation and treatment. Sometimes the fetal heartbeat is within the normal range but shows a troublesome pattern on the monitor sheet.

Non-reassuring fetal heartbeats are sometimes referred to as fetal distress. Fetal distress is thought to be caused by a temporary reduction of oxygen to the fetus, usually during a contraction. Factors that may contribute to fetal distress are:

- umbilical cord compression (squeezing) by uterine contraction
- umbilical cord prolapse (coming out ahead of baby)
- mother's blood pressure too high (preeclampsia)
- mother's blood pressure too low (drug or epidural reaction)
- maternal hemorrhage (placental abruption, placenta previa, trauma)
- maternal fever or infection of uterus and fetal membranes
- postdated pregnancy (old and calcified placenta)
- meconium or stress

How fetal distress is managed depends on several issues: whether the distress is mild or severe, how far the cervix is dilated, and whether the reason for the distress can be alleviated. For example, if the distress is mild and the cervix is fully dilated, the patient may be given oxygen and watched vigilantly with the plan that she will deliver soon. On the other hand, if the distress is severe and the cervix is many hours away from delivery, a C-section may be recommended. If the distress is severe and the cervix is fully dilated, an instrumented (forceps or vacuum) vaginal delivery may be an option. Your doctor will discuss these issues and options should fetal distress occur.

4. When would a vacuum or forceps be used during delivery?

A *vacuum* device is a small plastic cup that fits over the top of the baby's head and is attached to vacuum suction. Forceps are two metal, spoon-like instruments that are placed on either side of the baby's head. The doctor applies a steady pressure on the forceps. Both of these instruments were designed to help guide the baby's head out of the pelvis. They may be used when the mother cannot push the baby out by herself. She may not be able to push effectively because of exhaustion or (rarely) numbness due to an epidural. Or perhaps she is in the process of early pushing, but due to fetal distress, the baby needs to be delivered urgently.

Most pregnant women say that they prefer no vacuum or forceps with their delivery. Just about everyone agrees that it is preferable for the mother to have a natural and normal delivery, without the use of instruments. However, after several hours of pushing or in the case of fetal distress, an instrumented delivery may become a reasonable option. It's very important for your doctor to explain the situation to you along with the pros and cons of your options. As long as you and the baby are not in danger, your options are open. If fetal distress plays a factor, then a decision must be made quickly. Sometimes an instrumented delivery is attempted in the hope of avoiding a C-section. On occasion, mother and doctor will agree to forego the instrumented delivery attempt and proceed directly with a C-section.

More and more, C-sections seem to be replacing the instrumented (vacuum or forceps) delivery. This trend is due to several factors. Instruments could potentially cause damage to the baby. Also, these instruments require considerable training and skill to use properly. Many residency programs do not provide training in instrumented deliveries, especially forceps. In light of the medical and legal environment, many practitioners prefer to perform a C-section instead of using a vacuum or forceps. Talk with your doctor about his or her training and thoughts on these issues.

5.   Can my partner cut the baby's umbilical cord?

If things are going well, the delivering practitioner almost always encourages the dad or partner to cut the umbilical cord. Many new fathers are nervous about this. (Encourage them to do it anyway, because this may be a once-in-a-lifetime opportunity.) You may want to have a friend or family member take a picture or video of the cord-cutting event. It's a great keepsake.

In most deliveries there is no urgency to clamp and cut the cord. Therefore, the doctor has ample time to help your spouse or partner with this procedure. However, as mentioned earlier, in the case of fetal distress, thick meconium, or other urgent medical problems, the cord will be clamped and cut immediately. The spouse or partner may not be able to cut the cord because of the urgency of the situation. In the case of a C-section, it is likely that the spouse or partner may not be permitted to cut the cord because of the sterile field on the operating table.

17

After the Delivery

Congratulations! You're a mom! Simply amazing, isn't it? So much activity is swirling around you—holding and feeding your baby for the first time, receiving flowers and baby gifts, seeing relatives race to the nursery. At first it may be hard to get a moment to yourself to gather your thoughts. But enjoy this atmosphere of care and support because your hospital stay probably will last only one or two days.

Don't be surprised if it seems everyone is paying more attention to the baby than to you! Of course, you're important too, but modern medicine has a great way of helping nature to make sure your newborn is getting the best care possible.

Even with all the excitement, serious questions still need to be addressed. During your last trimester visits, the doctor may have encouraged you to start thinking about decisions to be made regarding circumcision, umbilical cord preservation, and the primary method you'll use to feed your baby. In fact, the advantages and disadvantages of each choice may have been on your mind for months. Now that you've delivered, your decisions will help determine some of the first actions to be taken to ensure the health and well-being of your precious new child.

1. What happens after my baby has been delivered?

Once delivered, your baby is usually placed on your abdomen. (Exceptions occur if some form of distress is present that requires medical attention. Another exception occurs if you specifically request that the baby not be placed upon your abdomen until he or she has been cleaned up, as some women prefer.) Within moments, the umbilical cord is clamped and cut. While still on your abdomen, the baby is placed in a warmed blanket and briskly scrubbed dry. This serves to dry and warm the baby and also causes the baby to cry, which opens the lungs and ensures good breathing movement. The baby stays with you during this entire time. Only in very rare cases is the baby whisked away to the nursery for further medical attention during this time.

Many women are surprised when they see their babies for the very first time. Newborn babies often have irregularly shaped heads and puffy eyes because of the molding required to fit through your birth canal. There may also be some bruising. Rest assured that within the next twenty-four to forty-eight hours, your baby's appearance will change remarkably for the better. Many babies are covered with a creamy white coating called *vernix*. It served as protection for their skin against the fluid environment within your uterus. It easily wipes clean.

Many babies, both male and female, are born with swollen genitals because of your increased hormones during pregnancy. The baby's genitals will return to normal within a few days.

Identification bands with your name are placed on both the baby's wrist and ankle. They match the wristband that you are given which will be your access to the nursery. An additional wristband is given to your spouse or partner.

Within the first hour after delivery, the nursery staff will place an antibiotic ointment in the baby's eyes to prevent infection, and will also weigh the baby. In most cases, a portable scale will be rolled into your labor and delivery room. Try to remember to take a picture of baby's first weigh-in. It's a momentous photo opportunity and keepsake.

Meanwhile, your doctor has been busy delivering your placenta and repairing any lacerations or episiotomy. He or she may request your help to push and deliver the placenta. Your doctor will also let you know about any stitches placed. (Don't worry; they dissolve and will not need to be removed at a later date.) Your bed is then placed back together and you are free to enjoy your new baby. Many women use this time to call friends and family members, attempt to breast-feed, and most of all, get acquainted with their beautiful new babies!

2. How is my newborn's health evaluated?

Apgar scores were designed by an anesthesiologist named Virginia Apgar. She invented this system as a uniform way of evaluating the well-being of newborn babies. The nursery staff assigns the scores as they evaluate five important organ systems of the newborn baby. The first assessment takes place at one minute after birth, and the second occurs five minutes after birth. Each of the five areas receives 0, 1, or 2 points; therefore, the total score is always between 0 and 10. The higher the score, the better the physical condition of the baby. Parents can learn the Apgar scores by checking with the nurse or nursery staff. These scores become a part of the baby's chart.

Scores above 7 are considered good. Babies almost never receive scores of 10. The one-minute score is sometimes artificially low due to fetal distress, meconium suction, or other resuscitation efforts. The five-minute score is considered more indicative of the baby's overall health and physical condition.

These scores become part of the baby's medical record. They indicate the nature of the baby's physical condition at the time of birth and provide valuable information to the nursery staff and the baby's pediatrician.

The Apgar Scoring System

System evaluated	0	1	2
Heart rate	Absent	Fewer than 100 beats per minute	More than 100 beats per minute
Breathing	None	Weak, irregular	Regular
Reflexes	None	Some	Sneeze, cough, grimace
Muscle tone	Limp	Some	Good flexion of arms
Color	Blue, pale	Body pink, hands and feet	Pink

3. Should we consider banking some of baby's umbilical cord blood?

Blood that is found in your baby's umbilical cord is rich in *stem cells*. Stem cells are "master cells" that are able to produce other cells found in the blood and immune systems. These cells can be easily collected at the time of delivery and cryo-preserved (freezing technique), in case they are needed later in life. These cells may substitute for a bone marrow transplant for diseases such as leukemia, certain forms of anemia, sickle cell disease, and certain types of cancer. The cells may be useful in treating other diseases in the future. Naturally, the blood is a guaranteed match for your baby. It also has about a 1 in 4 chance of being a match for a sibling.

This is a personal decision based on your beliefs, finances, and family medical history. Health care workers have become more familiar with cord blood banking and collection techniques. They are able to assist and advise you with your decision.

Cord Blood Banking

Advantages	Disadvantages
Easy and not painful to collect	Expensive, about $1,000 initial fee
Guaranteed match for baby	Storage fee, about $150 per year
1 in 4 chance of match for sibling	Pay even if don't need or use it
Successful as bone marrow transplants	Collection kit must be brought to delivery
May be stored for decades	Many unknowns, fairly new practice (1988)

4. Should I breast-feed my baby?

Just about every health care worker agrees that breast milk contains the best nutrients for your baby. Breast milk is the standard that formulas are judged against. However, many outstanding infant formulas are currently available. These improved formulas also do an excellent job of providing the proper nutrients for your baby.

Most women choose to breast-feed, if only for a short period of time. However, some women do not wish to breast-feed at all, for personal reasons. Women who decide against breast-feeding sometimes report that they are hassled by nurses and other members of the health care team. That is a most unfortunate situation. It is the job of the health care worker to ensure that the patient is well educated on her choices, and then to respect whatever decision she makes.

Assuming that baby is doing well, alert, and ready to suck, most babies are ready for their first feeding within a few hours after delivery. Babies who are particularly small or large may need to be fed within the first one or two hours after delivery.

If you do choose to breast-feed, lactation consultants are available in the hospital to help you get started. You may also set up an appointment with them outside of the hospital, but this may be at your

Breast-feeding

Advantages	Disadvantages
Offers best nutrients available	Must avoid certain foods; spicy, alcoholic
Contains factors to decrease infection	Must avoid certain medications
Contains factors to decrease allergies	May pass viral infections to baby
Encourages bonding	May not have sufficient milk
Costs little or nothing	Causes cramping and pain initially as uterus gets smaller
Offers convenience	Leak milk if hear, see, think about baby
Enables uterus to go back to original size more quickly	Experience engorgement; tender, painful, blocked ducts; infection

own expense. Make sure that you consume 1,000 mg of dietary calcium per day and that you increase your daily calorie intake by 300 to 500 over your nonpregnant level. Continue to take your prenatal vitamin and eat a well-balanced diet. Also, remember to increase your fluid intake and remain very well hydrated. There is very little you need to do to prepare your breasts for breast-feeding. The "roughing up" of the nipples by rubbing them with a brush or towel is no longer recommended to prepare them for breast-feeding. However, a good oil or lubricant on your nipples along with a gentle massage may provide some comfort.

Working moms face an extra challenge—how to breast-feed while away from the baby. Many women purchase breast pumps, which enable them to store their breast milk. The frozen or refrigerated breast milk can be used by the baby's caregiver. Other women choose to breast-feed while at home and have the caregiver feed the baby formula while they are at work.

The decision is yours to make. The most important thing is that you are comfortable with your decision and that you and your baby remain healthy.

5. Can my baby stay in my room while I am in the hospital?

The answer almost always is yes. Check with your hospital to learn their policy. Most hospitals have recently adopted a rooming-in policy whereby the baby stays with you in the room during your entire hospital stay. Occasionally, however, it may be necessary to monitor the baby closely in the nursery. In that case, you would have twenty-four-hour access to the nursery to visit your baby. Also, if you have had a particularly long, difficult labor or a C-section, you may request that the nursery watch the baby for a few hours so that you may get some much-needed rest. You can always call for assistance if you need some time for yourself or require other additional assistance.

6. If it's a boy, should he be circumcised?

Circumcision is the removal of the foreskin that shields the head of the penis. To circumcise or not to circumcise is an eternally debated question. The American Academy of Pediatrics released its most recent opinion in 1999. It states that the benefits are not significant enough to recommend circumcision as a routine procedure. Parents are encouraged to make the best decision for their child based on the risks and benefits of circumcision. Parents should also take their own cultural, religious, and ethnic traditions into consideration.

If you decide to have your son circumcised, it should be done within the first few days after birth. A doctor, either the baby's pediatrician or your OB/GYN physician, performs the procedure. In certain cultural or religious settings, a specially trained religious person called a *mohel* performs the circumcision. The procedure takes only minutes to perform.

Circumcision

Advantages	Disadvantages
Easier to clean, improved hygiene	Not medically necessary
May look like dad's and the other kids'	Painful procedure
Less likely to get urinary tract infections	Surgical risks
Part of ancient cultural and religious ritual	

Today, pain relief is used more commonly than even ten years ago. A topical anesthetic is used; or a regional nerve block, an injection to numb the nerve fibers in the penile area, is given.

Once home, the parents should keep the area clean with soap and water. Then, apply petroleum jelly liberally to prevent the skin from sticking to the diaper. If redness, infection, or bleeding occurs, call your doctor. Typically, the area heals within one to two weeks.

Deciding whether to have this procedure performed is a very personal issue. Think about how the pros and cons will affect your son. Consult with your close family members and friends, the baby's doctor, and your religious leader. That way, you can make the best decision for you and your baby.

7. How long can I expect to be in the hospital?

This decision is ultimately up to you, your doctor, the baby's doctor, and your medical insurance carrier. Assuming that you and baby are doing well, most doctors prefer that you and the baby stay for at least twenty-four hours after the delivery. This allows for close hospital observation during this important postdelivery time. Many women wish to stay a day or two longer. Unfortunately, your insurance company may dictate the length of your hospital stay. Assuming you had a normal and uncomplicated vaginal delivery, your insurer may pay for only one or two nights. If there was a complication or you delivered by C-section, additional days are often medically necessary and should be paid for by your medical insurance.

On occasion, the mother may be discharged from the hospital before the baby is discharged. This most commonly occurs when the baby is premature and needs special or intensive care. Under these circumstances, ask your hospital about a "nesting" option. With nesting, the mother is officially discharged from the hospital, but is allowed to stay in a vacant room (free of charge) to be near her baby.

Glossary

A

afterbirth: the placenta and the pregnancy membranes that are delivered after the birth of a baby

alpha feto-protein plus blood test: a blood test offered to pregnant women at between 16 and 20 weeks to assist in determining baby's risk of an open neural tube defect or Down syndrome

amniocentesis: a procedure, using a long slender needle placed through a pregnant woman's abdomen and into her uterus, to obtain a sample of amniotic fluid for evaluation

amniotic fluid: the fluid that surrounds a baby in the mother's uterus

anemia: a condition caused by a low red blood cell count

Apgar score: a numbering system that assesses five important organ systems of the newborn baby, used to evaluate the baby's well-being

aspiration: breathing foreign matter into the lungs

B

bag of water: the membranes and amniotic fluid surrounding a baby in the uterus

benzoyl peroxide: a chemical used in many common acne medications

biophysical profile: a special type of ultrasound that examines an unborn baby's organ systems to determine fetal well-being

birthing room: the hospital room for labor and delivery of a baby

Braxton Hicks contractions: sometimes called false labor, contractions that are weak, irregular, and not associated with a change in the mother's cervix

breast pump: a manual or electrical device that is placed on the breast to extract breast milk

breech: fetal position in which the feet or buttocks are closest to the cervix0

C

C-section: see Cesarean section

Cesarean section: method of delivering the baby through an abdominal incision

cerclage: a thick suture placed around the cervix to strengthen a weak or incompetent cervix

certified nurse-midwife: a registered nurse trained in providing prenatal care and in delivering babies

cervical dilation: see dilation

cervix: the opening of the uterus

chorionic villus sampling (CVS): a procedure during which a straw-like tube is placed through the vagina and into the placenta to collect tissue for genetic evaluation

chromosomes: parts of the cell that contain genetic information

circumcision: the removal of the foreskin that shields the head of the penis

cold knife cone: a surgical procedure, using a scalpel, to remove a small wedge of the cervix

colposcope: a small microscope-like device used to view cells on the cervix

colostrum: the clear or yellowish fluid that leaks from a pregnant woman's breasts before she produces milk

condyloma: the growth of wart-like cells, caused by a virus, on female genitalia

contractions: extreme muscle cramping within the uterus; also known as labor pains or labor contractions

crowning: the stage of delivery in which the top of the baby's head is bulging from the mother's vagina

CVS: see chorionic villus sampling

D

D & C: see dilation and curettage

DES: diethylstilbestrol, a synthetic estrogen once given to pregnant women and associated with abnormalities in the reproductive tracts of their female fetuses

dilation: the expansion of the opening of the cervix

dilation and curettage: a procedure in which the cervix is dilated with a surgical instrument and the uterus is scraped (curettage) to empty or sample its contents

doptone: a device used to listen to a baby's heartbeat while it is still in the uterus

double setup: a hospital room in which preparations have been made for both a vaginal and C-section delivery, often used in high-risk situations

doula: from the Greek word meaning "woman helping woman," a trained layperson who supports a woman during labor and delivery

Down syndrome: a genetic abnormality that results in a baby being born with varying degrees of mental retardation and physical defects

due date: the date on which a baby is due

dysmaturity syndrome: a fetal condition characterized by a long, skinny body and wrinkled skin

E

ectopic pregnancy: a pregnancy that is located somewhere other than the uterus, most commonly found in the fallopian tubes; it always requires medical attention and cannot result in a viable baby

effacement: the thinning of the cervix as labor progresses

ejaculation: discharge of semen from the penis

embryo: early developing baby, in humans usually the first 10 weeks of pregnancy

encephalitis: infection of the brain tissues

epidural: an anesthetic injection given in the lower back that causes loss of sensation from the waist down

episiotomy: a surgical incision made between the vagina and rectum for the purpose of enlarging the outlet for delivery

F

fallopian tubes: the pair of tubes that connect the uterus to the ovaries

false labor: sometimes called Braxton Hicks contractions, contractions that are weak, irregular, and not associated with a change in the mother's cervix

FAS: see fetal alcohol syndrome

fetal alcohol syndrome (FAS): a newborn's condition, marked by mental retardation and various physical defects because the mother consumed alcohol during pregnancy

fetal distress: non-reassuring fetal heartbeat, often due to reduced oxygen to baby during labor

fetal monitor: a machine used to observe fetal heart activity

fetus: the developing baby after the first 10 weeks of pregnancy

first trimester: the first 13 weeks of pregnancy

Foley bulb: a small balloon-like device inserted into bladder to hold the urinary catheter in place

folic acid: a water-soluble B-vitamin that helps build healthy cells

forceps: large tongs or spoon-like instrument used to grasp the baby's head to assist in delivery

fraternal twins: two babies born at the same time who do not share identical genetic material

G

genetic testing: lab tests designed to evaluate genetic makeup

genital herpes: a sexually transmitted disease caused by the herpes simplex viruses type 1 (HSV-1) and type 2 (HSV-2)

genital warts: the growth of abnormal cells, caused by a virus, on female

genitalia

gestational diabetes: a condition in which pregnancy hormones cause an imbalance in the metabolism of sugar and insulin

gestational wheel: an apparatus used to calculate pregnancy due dates

Group B strep bacteria: a type of bacteria, which may be carried by a mother, that can cause harm to the newborn baby

H

hemolytic anemia: breakdown and destruction of red blood cells leading to serious illness or death

hemorrhoids: dilated veins and swollen tissue near the rectum

herpes: see genital herpes

HIV: human immunodeficiency virus, the virus that causes AIDS

I

identical twins: two same-sex babies born at the same time who share identical genetic material

implantation bleeding: small amount of bleeding that may occur when an early pregnancy implants into the uterus

incompetent cervix: a cervix that is too weak to support the weight of a growing pregnant uterus, often resulting in second trimester miscarriage

induction: to artificially start labor contractions

intrauterine growth retardation: also known as IUGR, a harmful condition in which a baby does not grow properly within the uterus due to compromised placental blood supply caused by smoking, drugs, or high blood pressure, or unknown factors.

K

Kegel exercises: exercises for controlling urinary leakage by strengthening the pelvic floor muscles

L

labor contractions: see contractions

laminaria: thin, twig-like device made of seaweed, which is moistened and inserted into the cervix, causing the cervix to dilate

laparoscope: a long, slender telescope-like device that can be inserted into the abdomen (often via the navel) to examine and operate on organs within the body

LEEP: a surgical procedure (loop electrosurgical excision procedure) using a special electrical loop to remove a small cone or wedge of the cervix

M

meconium: greenish fecal material inside the fetal intestines.

membrane stripping: a procedure done during a pelvic exam in which the examiner stretches the cervix and sweeps his or her fingers over the membranes for the purpose of inducing labor contractions

meningitis: infection of the spinal tissues

menses: menstrual period

methotrexate: a chemotherapeutic drug that is sometimes used to treat an ectopic pregnancy

midwife: a layperson who delivers babies

miscarriage: spontaneous pregnancy loss

Montgomery's tubercles: small raised bumps, caused by pregnancy hormones, often found on the nipples of pregnant women

morning sickness: nausea and vomiting typically associated with early pregnancy

mucus discharge: see mucus plug

mucus plug: mucus that formerly lined the cervix, secreted through the vagina

N

neural tube defect: an abnormal opening along the spine or brain that will likely cause serious mental and physical problems for a baby

O

OB/GYN physician: a doctor who specializes in the medical care of women, the delivery of babies, and the medical and surgical treatment of the female reproductive system

ovulation: the releasing of an egg from a woman's ovary, usually two weeks after last menses

oxytocin: a natural hormone released by the body, responsible for uterine contractions

P

Pap smear: a test to check for abnormal cells on the cervix

Pap test: see Pap smear

pediatrician: a doctor who specializes in the medical care of babies and children

pelvic exam: a two-part procedure to evaluate the pelvis; in the first part a device is placed within the vagina so that the examiner may view and evaluate tissues; for the second part, the examiner uses one or two fingers within the vagina and the opposite hand on the patient's lower abdomen in order to examine the pelvic organs

perineum: the area between the vagina and the rectum

Glossary

Pitocin: an artificial hormone used to induce labor by causing uterine contractions

placenta: structure made of soft tissues and blood vessels, attached to the inside of mother's uterus, which provides nourishment to a fetus via the umbilical cord

placenta previa: the partial or complete covering of the cervix by the placenta, blocking the baby from a vaginal delivery

placental abruption: the partial or complete tearing away of the placenta from the uterine wall

postpartum sterilization: a surgical procedure to sever the fallopian tubes after a baby has been born, for the purpose of permanent sterilization

preeclampsia: type of high blood pressure associated with pregnancy that is harmful to mother and baby; also called pretoxemia

pregnancy-induced hypertension: see preeclampsia

pretoxemia: see preeclampsia

premature labor: contractions and cervical dilation that occur before the last month of pregnancy

prenatal classes: classroom instructions that prepare parents for pregnancy and childbirth

prenatal visit: an office visit with a physician during which a pregnant woman and her unborn baby are evaluated

progesterone: a female sex hormone, secreted to prepare the endometrium for implantation during pregnancy

prostaglandin: a medication that may be used to induce labor

PUPP: pruritic urticarial papules and plaques of pregnancy—a skin syndrome, unique to pregnancy and characterized by red rash and intense itching

pushing phase: the stage of labor when the cervix is completely dilated and effaced and pushing may safely begin in order to deliver the baby

R

respiratory syncytial virus: also known as RSV, a virus that causes severe respiratory infections and pneumonia, especially in babies and young children

Rh factor: a protein substance that may or may not be present on the surface of human blood cells

RhoGAM: a drug that prevents a mother's immune system from attacking her baby's blood

rubella: also known as German measles, this virus can cause serious birth defects in a fetus

S

second trimester: the second thirteen weeks of pregnancy

septicemia: an infection of the bloodstream

sperm: organisms within male semen that fertilize female eggs

stages of labor: stages of delivering a baby—contractions, pushing, and delivery of the placenta

stem cells: specialized "master" cells that are able to produce other cells found in the blood and immune systems

sterilization: a surgical procedure that severs the fallopian tubes in a female or the vas deferens in a male for the purpose of preventing future pregnancies

steroids: synthetic hormone medication

stretch marks: scars, elongated thin lines in the tissues, caused by stretching skin during pregnancy

syphilis: a sexually transmitted disease caused by a bacterium called Treponema pallidum.

T

third trimester: the last thirteen weeks of pregnancy

three-dimensional ultrasound (3-D): an ultrasound that provides a more detailed and lifelike image of an unborn baby

toxoplasmosis: a parasitic infection that can seriously damage the brain and nervous system of a baby

transducer: a device, placed on the pregnant woman's uterus, that transmits an image of the baby to the ultrasound screen

triage unit: an area of the labor and delivery department found in some larger hospitals, where patients are evaluated before being either sent home or admitted to the hospital

trimester: one of three terms into which pregnancy is divided

tubal ligation: form of permanent sterilization by tying or cutting the fallopian tubes to prevent future pregnancies

tubal pregnancy: see ectopic pregnancy

twin pregnancy: a uterus that contains two babies

U

ultrasound: a procedure that uses ultrasonic waves to view a baby's anatomy and major organs while it is still in the uterus

umbilical cord: the cord that connects the fetus to the placenta, providing the fetus with nutrients and oxygen

umbilical cord banking: the collecting, freezing, and storing of baby's umbilical cord blood for the purpose of treating possible future diseases in this baby or its siblings

uterine rupture: the tearing apart of the uterus, leading to fetal distress and requiring an emergent C-section

uterus: also known as the womb, this female pelvic organ expands during pregnancy and holds the growing baby

V

vacuum: a small suction device used to grasp the baby's head and assist in delivery

vaginal birth after Cesarean section (VBAC): refers to a delivery in which the current baby is delivered vaginally but a previous baby was delivered by C-section

vaginal breech: delivery of a baby in which the feet or buttocks are delivered first instead of the baby's head

vaginal delivery: method of delivering the baby through the vagina, considered the standard manner

vaginal infection: a disease within the vagina usually caused by either yeast or bacteria

varicose veins: swollen or dilated veins, often in the legs and pelvic region of a pregnant woman, caused by the increasing weight and pressure of the pregnancy

VBAC: see vaginal birth after Cesarean section

vernix: (or Vernix Caseosa) a creamy white coating that serves as protection for the unborn baby's skin while it's within the fluid environment of the uterus

version: a procedure to flip the unborn baby from a breech position to a head-down position so that a vaginal delivery can be anticipated

W

written birth plan: a list of requests and desires a new mother writes expressing what she wishes to experience during the birth process

Index

Index

Index

location, 29
prenatal classes, 29
preparation for going, 124
teaching, 29
hospital stay, 154, 155
human papilloma virus, 91
human placental lactogen (HPL), 87

I

implantation bleeding, 40
incompetent cervix, 34, 66-68, 92
treatment options, 67, 68
ultrasound, 66
indigestion, 73, 74, 78
induction of labor, 108–110
infant car seat, 61
infection, 20, 107, 109
infertility, 39
insulin, 88
insurance coverage,
doctors, 13, 64
doula, 140
genetic testing, 24
hospital, 28, 154
midwives, 14, 15
postpartum sterilization, 30, 117
prenatal classes, 62
prenatal vitamins, 23
ultrasounds, 55, 57, 59
intercourse, 6, 49, 97
intrauterine growth retardation (IUGR), 9
intravenous (IV)
antibiotics, 127
hydration, 36
lines, 128
iron supplements, 23

K

Kegel exercises, 75, 76

L

labor, 121–155
contractions, 122, 131, 132
delivery of the placenta, 131, 132
diabetes, 111
false, 102, 103
induction, 108–110
preeclampsia, 111
premature, 49
pushing, 131, 132, 141
stage I, 131, 132
stage II, 132
stage III, 132
stages, 131, 132
laminaria, 109
laparoscope, 40
lifestyle changes, 8-9, 45–52
listeria, 11
loop electrosurgical excision procedure (LEEP), 91
low birth weight, 9, 10
lung infection, 93
lupus, 35

M

maternity birthing center, 62
meconium, 111, 133, 134, 144
treatment options, 134
medical history, 19, 20, 91
medications
to end tubal ligation, 40
over-the-counter (OTC), 45, 46
meditation, 78
membranes, 134-136
see also amniotic fluid
meningitis, 93, 94

Index

About the Author

Susan Pick Warhus, M.D. is a board-certified OB/GYN physician and cofounder of the largest all-female practice in Phoenix, Arizona. During her clinical practice, she delivered more than 3,000 babies. Dr. Warhus is a member of the American College of OB/GYN and the American Medical Association. Prior to obtaining her medical degree from the University of Arizona School of Medicine, she earned a master's degree in business administration from Arizona State University and worked in the pharmaceutical industry.

Dr. Warhus is now a full-time writer, speaker, and patient educator for women's health issues. Dr. Warhus can be reached through her Web site: www.askdoctorsusan.com.

Other Consumer Health Titles from Addicus Books

Visit our online catalog at www.AddicusBooks.com

Organizations, associations, corporations, hospitals, and other groups may qualify for special discounts when ordering more than 24 copies. For more information, please contact the Special Sales Department at Addicus Books. Phone (402) 330-7493.

Email: info@AddicusBooks.com

Please send:

_____copies of_____

(Title of book)

at $_____each   TOTAL: _____

Nebraska residents add 5% sales tax   _____

Shipping/Handling
$4.00 postage for first book.
$1.10 postage for each additional book   _____

TOTAL ENCLOSED: _____

Name _____

Address _____

City_____State_____Zip _____

☐ Visa   ☐ MasterCard   ☐ American Express

Credit card number _____Expiration date _____

Order by credit card, personal check or money order. Send to:

Addicus Books
Mail Order Dept.
P.O. Box 45327
Omaha, NE 68145
Or, order **TOLL FREE: 800-352-2873**
or online at
www.AddicusBooks.com